T0247821

SIR THOMAS BROWNE

My Reading

GAVIN FRANCIS

SIR THOMAS BROWNE

The Opium of Time

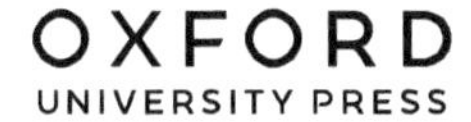

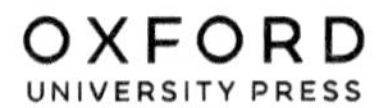

Great Clarendon Street, Oxford, OX2 6DP,
United Kingdom

Oxford University Press is a department of the University of Oxford.
It furthers the University's objective of excellence in research, scholarship,
and education by publishing worldwide. Oxford is a registered trade mark of
Oxford University Press in the UK and in certain other countries

Published in the United States of America by Oxford University Press
198 Madison Avenue, New York, NY 10016, United States of America

British Library Cataloguing in Publication Data
Data available

Library of Congress Control Number: 2022945388

ISBN 978–0–19–285817–7

DOI: 10.1093/oso/9780192858177.001.0001

Printed and bound by
CPI Group (UK) Ltd, Croydon, CR0 4YY

SERIES INTRODUCTION

This series is built on a simple presupposition: that it helps to have a book recommended and discussed by someone who cares for it. Books are not purely self-sufficient: they need people and they need to get to what is personal within them.

The people we have been seeking as contributors to *My Reading* are readers who are also writers: novelists and poets; literary critics, outside as well as inside universities, but also thinkers from other disciplines—philosophy, psychology, science, theology, and sociology—beside the literary; and, not least of all, intense readers whose first profession is not writing itself but, for example, medicine, or law, or a non-verbal form of art. Of all of them we have asked: what books or authors feel as though they are deeply *yours*, influencing or challenging your life and work, most deserving of rescue and attention, or demanding of feeling and use?

What is it like to love this book? What is it like to have a thought or idea or doubt or memory, not cold and in abstract, but live in the very act of reading? What is it like to feel, long after, that this writer is a vital part of your life? We ask our authors to respond to such bold questions by writing not conventionally but personally—whatever 'personal' might mean, whatever form or style it might take, for them as individuals. This does not mean overt confession at the expense of a chosen book or author; but nor should our writers be afraid of making autobiographical connections. What was wanted was whatever made for their own hardest thinking in careful relation to quoted sources and specifics. The work was to go on in the taut and resonant space between these readers and their chosen books. And the interest within that area begins precisely when it is no longer clear how much is coming from the text and how much is coming from its readers—where that distinction is no longer easily tenable because neither is sacrificed to the other. That would show what reading meant at its most serious and how it might have relation to an individual life.

Out of what we hope will be an ongoing variety of books and readers, *My Reading* offers personal models of what it is like to care about particular authors, to recreate through specific examples imaginative versions of what those authors and works represent, and to show their effect upon a reader's own thinking and development.

ANNE CHENG
PHILIP DAVIS
JACQUELINE NORTON
MARINA WARNER
MICHAEL WOOD

For scholars
who make their heads not graves,
but treasures of knowledge

also by Gavin Francis

True North: Travels in Arctic Europe
Empire Antarctica: Ice, Silence & Emperor Penguins
Adventures in Human Being
Shapeshifters: A Doctor's Notes on Medicine & Human Change
Island Dreams: Mapping an Obsession
Intensive Care: A GP, a Community, & a Pandemic
Recovery: The Lost Art of Convalescence

CONTENTS

CHRONOLOGY OF DR THOMAS BROWNE'S LIFE, 1605–1682

1605—	Born 19 October in Cheapside, London, the son of a silk merchant
1613—	His father, Thomas Browne Sr. dies. His mother Anne Garaway remarries
1616—	August 20 admitted for 'grammar study' at Winchester College
1623—	Travels in Ireland with his stepfather, Sir Thomas Dutton
1623—	December 5 matriculates at Broadgates Hall, Oxford, to study arts
1627—	January 31 graduates BA
1629—	June 11 graduates MA, and begins to study medicine
1631—	Moves to Montpellier, a medical school famed for botany
1632—	Moves to Padua, a medical school famed for anatomy
1633—	Moves to Leiden, a medical school famed for Protestant piety and bedside teaching, where he is awarded an M.D. (his thesis is on smallpox)
1634—	Moves to Halifax, begins work as a physician
1635 (approx)—	Writes ***Religio Medici***, for distribution among friends

1637—	Settles in Norwich and begins to expand his medical practice
1641—	Is married to Dorothy Mileham
1642—	Unofficial editions of ***Religio Medici*** become so popular that Browne is obliged to issue an approved edition
1644—	A son, Edward, is born, who goes on to become King's physician, and president of the Royal College of Physicians. There will be nine more children, four of whom will survive to adulthood.
1646—	First edition of ***Pseudodoxia Epidemica*** or ***Vulgar Errors*** published. It will go through many editions, his most popular book in his lifetime
1658—	***Garden of Cyrus / Urne Buriall*** published together—meditations on death and vitality, funereal practices as well as patterns in nature
1662—	Is asked to give an opinion at a witch trial in Bury St Edmunds. The accused women, Amy Denny and Rose Cullender, are hanged
1671—	Is knighted when Charles II visits Norwich. The honour was initially intended for the mayor who, as a parliamentarian, had declined
1682—	Dies October 19, his birthday, aged 77
1716—	***Christian Morals***, a collection of previously unpublished late meditations on the practical application of faith, is published posthumously
1723—	Various other posthumous works are published, including ***Museum Clausum*** and ***Letter to a Friend***

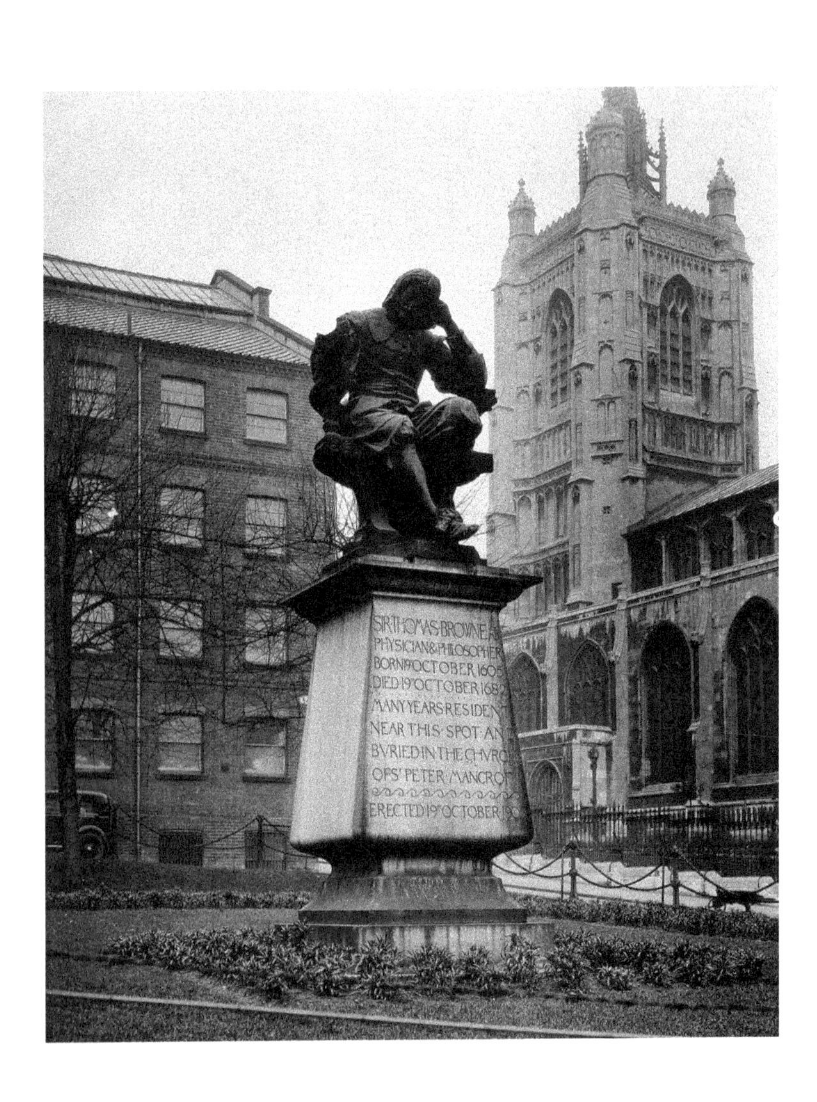
SIR THOMAS BROWNE
PHYSICIAN & PHILOSOPHER
BORN 19 OCTOBER 1605
DIED 19 OCTOBER 168
MANY YEARS RESIDEN
NEAR THIS SPOT AN
BVRIED IN THE CHVRC
OF S. PETER MANCRO
ERECTED 19 OCTOBER 19

AN INTRODUCTORY LETTER TO DR BROWNE

Dear Dr Browne,

We are separated by three and half centuries, and by faith, geography, classical learning, social status, and much else besides. Both of us have worked as general medical practitioners and as writers, but your career through Winchester, Oxford, and the elite universities of Europe sets us apart. You'd perhaps scarcely believe that by the twentieth century a Scot like me, educated at a comprehensive school that was open to all, would be paid by the state to train as a doctor and qualify into a medical system that offers treatment *gratis* to the patient, according to need rather than demand. In your age most Scots were obliged to travel to Dutch universities for their medical education because, though they shared your king, they didn't share your church.

Characteristic of your genius is a phrase in which you describe your intention to embark upon a 'cosmography of my self'. It's a phrase both celestial and personal, expansive and expressive of your restless curiosity, of an attitude that looks with tenderness at the human condition, yet with ambition at human potential. Your work as a physician amply provided you with evidence of just how much wonder is to be found in human anatomy and physiology, in individual patients' resilience, as well as proof of the fragility of life. 'I, that have examined the parts of man, and know upon what tender filaments that fabric hangs, do wonder that we are not always so; and considering the thousand doors that lead to death, do thank my God that we can die but once.' Average human life expectancy doubled over the course of the twentieth century, and as a consequence, far more of my patients have the opportunity to die old in their beds than yours ever did. But the revelations of biochemistry and physiology enjoyed by my own age make it seem to me *more* rather than less astonishing that life carries on.

Just as there is a great deal that separates us, there is a great deal that I suspect we have in common. Though I didn't share your classical education, we do share a fundamental curiosity about the world and about people—what motivates and inspires their ambitions, how they see their lives and how they attempt to navigate the many paths towards happiness. There's no better profession than medicine for seeing how those paths turn out—for good and for bad. Your love for what is often now called 'the natural world'—for you, the *whole* world—offered you ample evidence of the munificence of your God, as well as an apparently limitless source of inspiration and contemplation.

You wrote books on faith, on the limits of knowledge, on vitality and mortality, on patterns in nature, on what constitutes a good life. Your writings on the confounding issue of money in medicine lead me to suspect that you'd be a supporter of the kind of health service your own country now enjoys. No record survives of which of the Hippocratic writings you were questioned on for your MD thesis, but I like to imagine that you were asked about those ones that resonate with the pragmatic compassion and humanitarianism evident everywhere in your writing: 'It is better to reproach a patient that you have saved than to extort money from those who are at death's door', or 'For where there is love of man, there is also love of the art.' I wonder what you'd have said of the news that smallpox, the subject of your thesis, would by my own age be eradicated. The survival rates for infants and young children have in my own age been utterly transformed; you lost five of your children to diseases you thought of with fatalism and prayer, but which I am lucky enough to think of as treatable conditions, defeated thanks to a scientific method that you witnessed at its birth.

Your many books, and in particular *Religio Medici*, were first brought to my attention because they were admired by Sir William Osler, a renowned humanitarian physician of the later nineteenth century who loved your humility, your curiosity, and your sense of wonder. It was thanks to Osler that I began to read your own work, grateful to recognize among some of your own attitudes to the practice of medicine a few of my own.

I have read that your knighthood was accidental, in that the intended recipient, a Parliamentarian Mayor of Norwich, declined the honour when Charles II came to the city. You received the honour instead, through the expedient of being the most esteemed member of the community that happened to be close at hand. But for almost the entirety of your adult life you were simply 'Dr Browne', and though your family were prosperous, and your father a silk merchant, you didn't come from nobility.

Your letters to your son lament the cost of the christenings and burials you paid out for your dead children, of the pressures of running your large household, the challenge of being able to offer free 'physic' to the poor while maintaining an income of £1000 a year, and taking care not to give in to greed. 'Of that subterraneous idol and god of the earth' you wrote of gold, 'I do confess I am an atheist.' Yet you pushed your son Edward to succeed, and enter that stratum of high society which takes means for granted.

Those writings of yours that survive are all but silent on the injustice of the English colonial project then evolving in Ireland, though you saw the consequences of that brutal process first-hand on a tour with your stepfather. You thought your faith should spread over the globe, replacing all other spiritual traditions. Perhaps because of your adherence to the Bible as truth you remained convinced to the last that witchcraft was real, and did little to prevent the conviction of accused women who, whatever their crimes, surely cannot have had supernatural powers. But there's enough doubt in what survives of your testimony to suggest that you too had suspicions of the innocence of women accused of witchcraft, and that you would have questioned the justice of your countrymen's meddling in Ireland. You served the poor of Norwich, you roundly rejected anti-Semitism (carefully listing all the ways in which English prejudices against Jews were unfounded), and you worked tirelessly to reveal common errors in folk belief. All these actions imply a freedom from prejudice that many could do well to learn from today.

To open your book *Vulgar Errors* at random is to be offered a glimpse of the breadth of your curiosities. The nature of pigmies; the medicinal power of unicorn horns; the existence of mermaids, whether Adam or Eve had navels; the flux of the Nile; why the smoke of sulphur is white; what is augured by rainbows. You were never afraid to leave your conclusions vague, unfinished, or declare yourself unable to decide. Your authorities tend to be classical or scriptural—you mourned the loss of the glory years of Muslim scholarship—but just as often you showed yourself to be what we'd now call a 'scientist', by testing out ideas for yourself. You wrote of hanging kingfishers from threads of 'untwisted silk' to prove that they do not indicate the direction of the wind; of prodding your own eye when 'beholding a Candle' to prove that a disturbance in alignment creates the illusion of double vision.

Though the majority of your life was spent settled in a Norwich medical practice, you never lost the love of travel that saw you tour Ireland and Europe, and edit your son Edward's travel journals. For me, a telling and delightful detail of your love of travel lies in a list that has survived of those books read to you in your old age by your daughter Betty: travel accounts of China, Turkey, Naples, Venice; Abel Tasman's voyage to Terra Australis; Rycaut's writings on the Turkish sultans.

Travel is easier now, and many of those journeys you were able only to read of I have made, not only as a traveller but as a physician. You were in many respects a quintessential Englishman who wrote of his church and his nation with pride, but you were also a consummate European, repeating with satisfaction how many of that continent's languages your books had been translated into, and who journeyed between Italy, France, and the Netherlands to complete your own medical training. In the pages that follow I hope to reflect on the experience of following in your footsteps to Leiden and Padua in particular.

But your project, at heart, has always seemed to me to have been one of humanity and humanitarianism, an enquiry facilitated by your work as a general physician in a provincial city practice.

In *Religio Medici* you wrote of the glories that can be experienced through travel, but also of a belief very close to my own motivations and enthusiasms: the miraculous nature of life, and in particular human life, in which life becomes conscious of itself. 'The whole creation is a mystery, and particularly that of man', you wrote. In the three and a half centuries since your own time, many aspects of nature that were mysteries to your contemporaries have been explained by science. Much, though, remains poorly understood: humanity is not a great deal further forward in understanding one of the greatest enigmas—the emergence of conscious experience—than it was in your own time.

You did not perhaps imagine that four centuries after your birth we'd still be reading you: 'Men's works have an age like themselves', you wrote, 'and though they outlive their authors, yet have they a stint and period to their duration.' We *are* still reading you, though with every decade the transformations of the English language render your own prose more challenging. In the following essays I'll be careful to transcribe your writings with accuracy in your choice of words, but will bring in my own age's conventions of spelling. I hope this will better convey to the reader the power of your words, while retaining the idiosyncrasies of your prose.

For all the changes in human society over the last four centuries your works remind me to attend to the now—to the only world I'll ever know—and to work with diligence on my own curiosities and enthusiasms, pursuing the great and timeless questions that recur in every age. Yours was a time in which the alchemical enquiries of the Middle Ages were slowly giving way to a more rigorous scientific method. I intend the essays that follow to perform an alchemy of their own, bubbling together stories from your life and your fascinations with my reflections as a twenty-first-century writer and doctor, so that we can see what new alloys, tinctures, and solutions might result. The word 'render' can mean to portray, to yield, to restore, and to lay out a matter before others. I've thought of this book as a 'rendering' rather than an orthodox biography because it aims to render the value of your life, your work, and your books.

Yours, etc.

Dr Gavin Francis

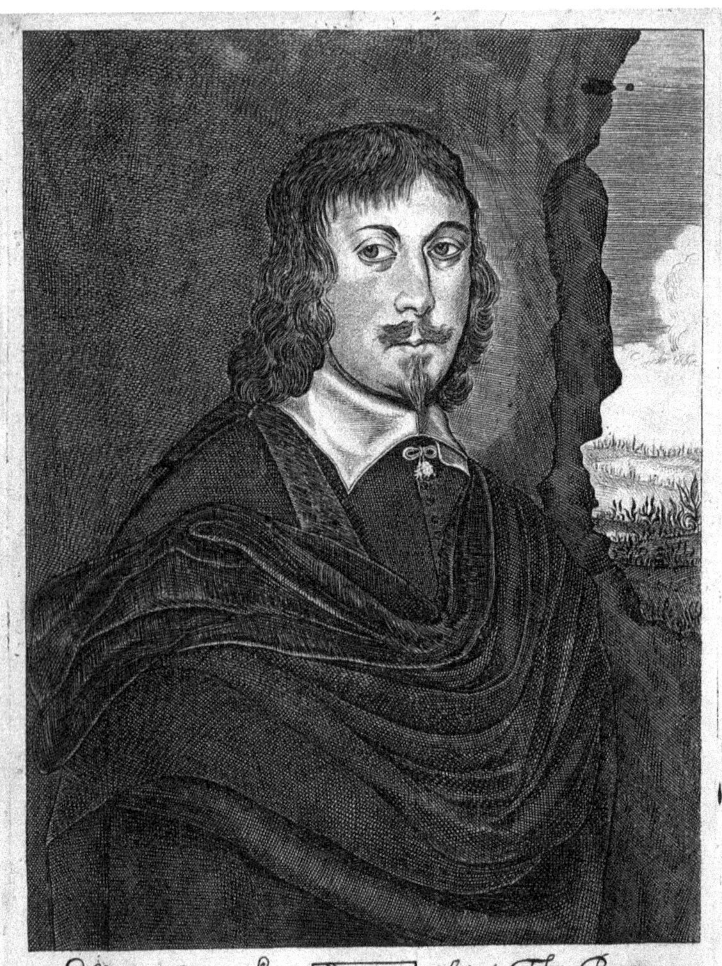

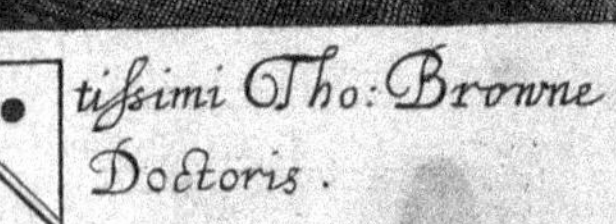

Effigies Viri doc= tissimi Tho: Browne Med: Doctoris.

1

AMBIGUITY

> Browne's style, intricate, opulent, performed with tweezers and microscope, describes a malleable prose, in whose minutiae, every object, and each twist of the pen has theological purpose.
>
> Kevin Killeen, *Thomas Browne: Selected Writings*

> The fallacy of equivocation... which conclude from the ambiguity of some one word, or the ambiguous syntaxis of many put together...
>
> *Vulgar Errors*, Bk 1 Ch. 4

In the Medical Hall of Padua's old university, upstairs in the *Palazzo Bo*, there are glass cabinets containing the skulls of long-dead professors. Students still defend their theses surrounded by these skulls, and observed by flayed reproduction figures from the Flemish anatomist Vesalius's great masterpiece of utilitarian anatomy, *On the Fabric of the Human Body*, researched and written in Padua, and published in 1543. Galen, the authority in anatomy for over a millennium, had learned some of his knowledge through working as a physician to gladiators of the city of Pergamon in Asia Minor, but most of it was gleaned through the dissection of Barbary apes and other mammals. Vesalius recognized that a great deal of Galen's anatomy was wrong, and using bodies pulled down from gibbets and the noose, he revolutionized what constituted authority. Vesalius taught in makeshift, impromptu anatomy theatres, but in 1594 a permanent one was built and the oldest still extant. In Padua I stood at the base of its elliptical, inverted cone; seat rows climbed heavenwards from the slab where cadavers were once dismembered, like contours in a map of a quarry hole, or the bolgias of Dante's notorious plan of Hell.

In Padua's adjacent *Sala dei Quaranta,* or Hall of the Forty, Galileo's wooden podium is still venerated. It looked like a pulpit from the protestant churches of my youth; the tour guide told me that Galileo's lectures were the best attended of any teacher of the seventeenth century, and that his eighteen years in Padua were the happiest of his life. Like Vesalius, as a challenger to received truths he found sanctuary in the Venetian republic. The 'forty' portraits on the walls were those of foreigners who had studied in Padua and gone on to change the way medicine was practised in their home countries, or even more widely across Europe. Among the portraits, I made out Harvey, Lineacre, Rudbeck, Capodistria. No sign, of course, of Browne. Browne's fame in medical matters never extended far beyond Norwich, no matter how far his fame would spread among lovers of books and of literature.

In the *Aula Magna,* or Great Hall, Galileo's face was one of four that peered down from the ceiling like the four evangelists, or medallions of the four rightly guided caliphs. The walls were encrusted with heraldic crests and stiff, bearded portraits, emblematic of the kind of seeking after immortality that Browne would mock as so senseless in *Urn Burial.* And the effect of all these authorities bearing down was unexpected. Rather than inspirational, as was presumably their intent, they became cloying, claustrophobic, deadening.

On the way down the stairs another statue was pointed out—the only one of a woman. The guide told my group how Elena Lucrezia Cornaro Piscopia was, in 1678, Italy's first woman graduate after successfully defending her thesis and being duly awarded a degree in philosophy. The subject matters in which she dealt concerned theology, not philosophy, but as a woman, the degree of theology was barred to her.

From the Palazzo Bo I walked south, past an old Franciscan hospital, through the ghetto, past the city cathedral, to reach the botanical gardens, established in 1545. These are among the oldest medicinal gardens still in use, on the same site that Browne knew. It's a World Heritage Site, described by UNESCO like this:

> It preserves its original layout, a circular central plot symbolizing the world surrounded by a ring of water representing the ocean. The plan is a perfect circle with a large inscribed square, which is subdivided into four units by orthogonal paths, oriented according to the main cardinal directions. When the four entrances were redesigned in 1704, the wrought-iron gates leading to the inner circles and the four acroteria were placed on eight pillars and surmounted by four pairs of wrought-iron plants. During the first half of the 18th century, the balustrade, which runs along the top of the entire 250 m of the circular wall, was completed. The Botanical Garden of Padua houses two important collections: the library that contains more than 50,000 volumes and manuscripts of historical and bibliographic importance and the herbarium, which is the second most extensive in Italy. Particularly rare plants were also traditionally collected and grown in the garden. Currently, there are over 6,000 species, arranged according to systematic, utilitarian and ecological-environmental criteria, as well as thematic collections.[1]

The square of the gardens sits nested within a circular arrangement representing the world just as Vitruvius described, and Leonardo da Vinci realized, the perfect symmetry of the human form conforming to both square and circle. A runnel of water lay in a sweeping curve around the circular elements of the garden, the way Homer and Herodotus imagined Oceanus surrounding the habitable earth.

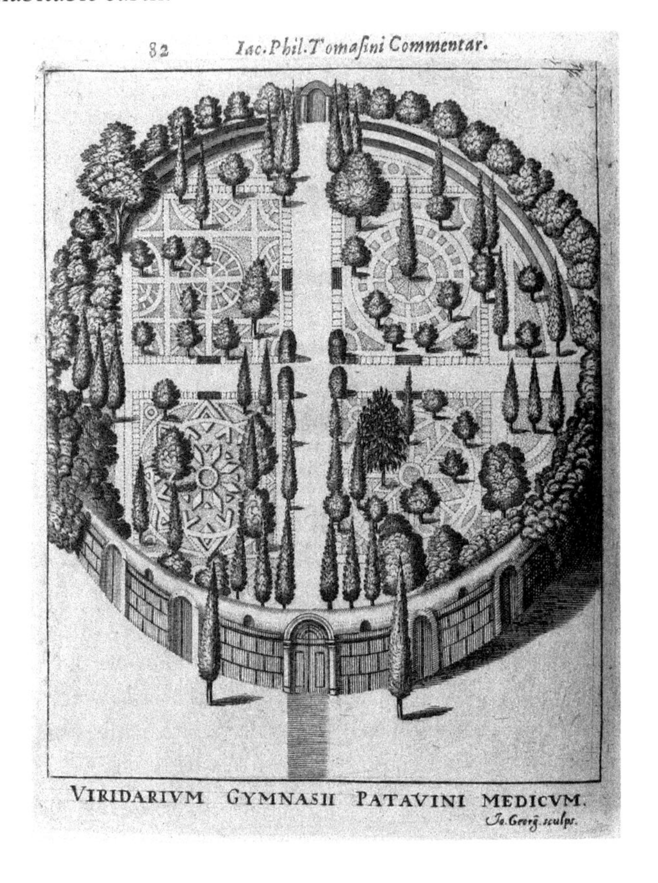

VIRIDARIVM GYMNASII PATAVINI MEDICVM.

On those curving paths between medicinal plants gathered from across the globe—gingko and magnolia, orchids and succulents—and among smells of jasmine and the sound of bird-song, I met with a palm tree planted in the 1580s, and now pressed up against the walls of its own glasshouse. When it was already two hundred years old, Goethe wrote about the qualities of this palm, in his 'Essay on the Metamorphosis of Plants'. Despite its venerable age and robust quality, the aspect of the palm that appealed to Goethe was the way its leaves began as continuous across their breadth, but progressively feathered into frayed leaflets without losing any of their function. There's no record of what Browne made of the palm, which would have been only forty or fifty years old when he studied the medicinal plants of the garden. He would have enjoyed knowing that it would live on into the deep future of our own time: 'generations pass while some trees stand', he wrote in *Urn Burial*, 'and old families last not three oaks.'[2] Five centuries old, the palm was still reproducing—a veritable tree of life.

*

In this city of great medical authorities, ancient gardens, pomp and pride in tradition, of the right way and wrong way of doing things, I wonder how Browne dealt with his innate capacity to be at ease with ambiguity, and reside in mystery. He was curious about everything, but also content not to know. He never took a shortcut to a conclusion when he could take a perambulation; he never leapt to a certainty when he could dwell for a while in enigma. Circumlocutions are his defining style, and he prefers to avoid being pinned down to categorical statements ('I am half of the opinion…'; 'I could easily believe…'). Samuel Johnson said of this tendency:

> His exuberance of knowledge, and plenitude of ideas, sometimes obstruct the tendency of his reasoning, and the clearness of his decisions: on whatever subject he employed his mind, there started up immediately so many images before him, that he lost one by grasping another. His memory supplied him with so many illustrations,

> parallel or dependent notions, that he was always starting into collateral considerations: but the spirit and vigour of his persuit always gives delight; and the reader follows him, without reluctance, thro' his mazes, in themselves flowery and pleasing, and ending at the point originally in view.[3]

This love of ambiguity and uncertainty, obscurity and opacity, is surely part of the reason Browne isn't remembered on the walls of Padua's *Sala dei Quaranta,* and is perhaps also related to the reason that he never became a Fellow of the Royal Society. But that love is just as equally the reason why many still read him. Francis Bacon made an immeasurably greater contribution to modernity by laying the foundations to the scientific method, but is read now almost exclusively by historians of science and of philosophy, not enthusiasts of literature. '[T]he universe to the eye of the human understanding is framed like a labyrinth', wrote Bacon,[4] 'presenting as it does on every side so many ambiguities of way, such deceitful resemblances of objects and signs, natures so irregular in their lines, and so knotted and entangled. and then the way is still to be made by the uncertain light of the sense.' He worried that human reason would prove insufficient to untangle the mysteries of nature, and that only through the development of a new rigorous and scientific approach would the hidden workings of nature be revealed: '[T]he state of knowledge is not prosperous nor greatly advancing ... a way must be opened for the human understanding entirely different from any hitherto known.'

But Browne wasn't ultimately interested in exploring new modes 'different from any hitherto known'; he was interested in the classics, in scripture, and the plants and animals of his own back yard. When the evidence of those sources contradicted one another, he shrugged, smiled, made a note, and turned the page.

*

That he revels in inconsistency, resides in ambiguity, and easily rests in paradox, is one of the defining features of Browne's prose. Virginia Woolf thought that it was this quality of indecision that 'paved the way for all psychological novelists, autobiographers, confession-mongers, and dealers in the curious shades of our private life'.[5] He 'brings the remote and the incongruous astonishingly together', floated high over the absurdities of human life, only to descend abruptly, without warning, to examine some peculiarity of his own experience. 'In short, as we say when we cannot help laughing at the oddities of people we admire most, he was a character', Woolf wrote, 'and the first to make us feel that the most sublime speculations of the human imagination are issued from a particular man, whom we can love.' In her essay *Personalities,* Woolf wrote that it was those writers who are 'elusive, enigmatic, impersonal' that she most admired, whose lives were less interesting than their books, because it was into their books that everything of value was distilled.

From his books you would hardly know that Browne lived through the ferocious years of the English Civil War. 'You might read every word', wrote Alexander Whyte, 'and never discover that a sword had been unsheathed or a shot fired in England all the time he was living and writing there ... Sir Thomas Browne would seem to have possessed all the political and religious liberty he needed.'[6] Though a royalist by temperament and conditioning, he never explicitly took sides—wise perhaps for a physician the majority of whose patients were sympathetic to Cromwell, but also characteristic of someone who wrote at the beginning of his writing career, 'I have no genius to disputes in religion',[7] and of Roman Catholics, 'we have reformed from them, not against them.'[8] Whyte adored this quality in Browne: 'He does not unchurch or ostracise any other man'; 'He has never been able to alienate or exasperate himself from any man whatsoever because of a difference of an opinion.'[9] This wavering is entirely consistent with his reason; I imagine him shaking his head in pity and in sadness at the polarization of opinion now generated by the widespread use of social media feeds, funded by advertising, that are tailored to maximize engagement irrespective of content. 'But the mortalest enemy unto knowledge, and that which has done the greatest execution upon truth, has been a peremptory adhesion unto authority', he wrote.[10] If Hippocrates, Galen, and Aristotle could admit when they were wrong, how can anyone else ever state their beliefs with certainty? And Browne's readers should open his books conscious that nothing written there is beyond dispute: the words, he said, should be understood as mere opinions, 'nor have we Dictator-like obtruded our conceptions.'[11] This is one of the most Montaignesque passages in Browne, who wrote 'these are but my humours and opinions, and I deliver them but to show what my conceit is, and not what ought to be believed.'[12] Even *Vulgar Errors*, the book that more than any others seeks to establish authoritative truths, begins by dismissing recourse to authority. Browne uses paradox as a way of getting closer to understanding rather than truth, because he believes logic and reason alone aren't enough for humanity to achieve a broader knowledge that includes a living faith. Paradox and contradiction assist his faith, they don't detract from it. He quotes Tertullian—'I believe because it is impossible'—and in Christian Morals he wrote that we should 'delight to be alone *and* single with omnipresency' (my italics).

*

Ambiguity allowed Browne to more closely reconcile an understanding of the world and humanity's place in it with his faith. He loved the classics, yet took nothing on authority, neither the distinguished Padovan professors of his youth, nor Galen, Hippocrates, or his beloved Aristotle. Ambiguity was also a way of flexing his literary muscles, building those elaborate, sumptuous, grandiloquent sentences. Woolf wrote that his books were the only ones she knew other than the Bible that made her feel like a congregation rather than a reader. He had no genius for disputes, he said, but he did have a genius for perseverance, for enquiry, for reconciliation and exposition of different sides of any argument. As a close reader of Ovid's *Metamorphoses*, he knew that all change is charged with potential for good and for ill, and he held this knowledge of uncertainties in trust for his patients. This is one way in which his talent for ambiguity was put in the service of his patients.

In a book about the history of vaccination, the American essayist Eula Biss wrote of the way an acceptance of ambiguity helped her appreciate the essence of the doctor–patient relationship. As a mother, society urged her to 'trust' her instincts, but in matters such as vaccinology—the details of which specialists labour at for decades of their lives—she had little faith in her own ability to make the right choices: 'A trust', she wrote, '—in the sense of a valuable asset placed in the care of someone to whom it does not ultimately belong—captures, more or less, my understanding of what it is to have a child.'[13] She talks through the choice of whether or not to vaccinate with her own father, a physician, who tells her: 'If you're going to get good medical care, you're going to have to trust someone.' Trust is the central issue in any medical transaction, lamentably often characterized as paternalistic. For Biss, good trust makes paternalism unnecessary, and where there's no trust, paternalism is unconscionable. Her words reminded me of all the thousands of paediatric consultations I've had over twenty-five years of medical practice, some successful, some unsuccessful. In any consultation with a child, there's at least two patients. If you don't inspire trust in the child's parent, you've failed.

But being trustworthy necessitates being honest about the doubt inherent in so much of medicine. There are just too many variables at play in any illness, and even the most technomedical of modern encounters, armed with batteries of blood tests and scans, will never be able to gather enough data to provide certainty about all outcomes. Doctors recognize this and make their decisions based on an ever-shifting formula of test data, impressions, experience, and guesswork. The very best doctors do this while intuiting, in the space of a short encounter, what kind of physician the patient before them prefers. Is it someone who needs to hear reassurances and certainties—however unjustified? Or someone happy to embark on a collaborative conversation that acknowledges doubt and ambiguity, respectful of both partners' experience? This principle extends from the most simple clinical encounter—which cream to put on eczematous skin, which antibiotic to use in a urine infection—through to those urgent, devastating, but necessary conversations with patients (and their families) approaching the end of life. I was always taught that, in matters of end-of-life care, hope and realism can be irreconcilable if the facts of the matter are laid bare. Physicians have a responsibility to offer information to any patient that asks for it, but they also have the obligation to respect the patient's unjustified optimism, if that is the patient and their family's wish.

The kind of circumlocutions Browne excelled in can prove useful in these conversations, and it seems he indulged in them too, even in moments when he had resolved to be direct. 'Upon my first visit I was bold to tell them who had not let fall all hopes of his recovery', he wrote of his conversation with the family of Robert Loveday, who was dying of consumption (likely tuberculosis), 'that in my sad opinion he was not like to behold a grasshopper, much less to pluck another fig.'[14]

Kay Redfield Jamieson, a professor of psychiatry at Johns Hopkins University, suffers from a bipolar disorder that has occasioned oscillations in mood from suicidal despair to life-wrecking elation. Bipolar illness could be characterized as a condition in which the inherent ambiguity of life fades from view and is replaced by extreme swings of conviction. In her memoir about her illness, *An Unquiet Mind*, she wrote about encountering an ideal doctor who could provide an antidote to such dangerous certainty:

> He was at ease with ambiguity, had a comfort with complexity, and was able to be decisive in the midst of chaos and uncertainty. He treated me with respect, a decisive professionalism, wit, and an unshakeable belief in my ability to get well, compete, and make a difference.[15]

At first reading, Redfield Jamieson's description comes across as paradox: how can a clinician can offer certainty and 'unshakeable belief', but at the same time witticisms and an ease with ambiguity? Perhaps levity is the answer, holding certainties lightly, aware of absurdity. Laughter can be a great reconciler, a flag put down in a discussion to indicate a delicate moment, gauge potential responses, or cover up ambiguities as they arise. Browne was aware of its power, and how to use it carefully in conversation: 'For a laugh there is of contempt or indignation, as well as of mirth and jocosity.'[16] Sometimes a short laugh, as a response, allows a patient of mine to acknowledge they've heard something difficult to take in, and offers a pivot point in the development of a conversation—either partner can choose to take the laugh as the end point of a narrative thread, a turning point, or a new beginning.

It's my experience that doctors and their patients benefit when both acknowledge the degree of uncertainty in medical practice. Circumlocutions and elaborate metaphors are as necessary a part of a physician's toolkit as a stethoscope and tendon hammer; medical schools should perhaps teach William Empson's *Seven Types of Ambiguity* as closely as they teach the seven muscles of the calf.

*

There is one more element of Browne's wordplay which threatens to cancel out that focus on ambiguity which I so love, and that is his extreme adoration of the specificity of words. His logophilia was such that the English language of his day was often insufficient to his purposes, and he sought again and again to create utterly new coinages through his profound knowledge of the classics, particularly of Latin.

In a lecture to the Thomas Browne Society of Norwich (2018), the poet George Szirtes listed some of his favourites among the words Browne has left us:

> *medical, electricity, hallucination, inconsistent, migrant, ambidextrous, computer, coma, cryptography, ferocious, incisor, follicle, expectoration, antediluvian, circumstantially, presumably, traditionally, invariably, append, aquiline, biped, carnivorous, coexistence, compensate, exhaustion, indigenous, locomotion, misconception, prefix, pubescent, temperamental, veterinarian, typographer, deleterious*[17]

But it was the scrupulous research of Christopher Hitchings, in his doctoral research for University College London on the importance of Browne to Samuel Johnson, which first revealed to me the true extent of the debt owed by the English language to the works of Dr Browne. Hitchings searched Johnson's *Dictionary* by CD-ROM and found well over two thousand entries traced by Johnson to Browne, many of which seemed uniquely attributable to Browne, and of which only a tiny proportion had been wrongly connected to his books. For all that abundance, Browne is only the eleventh most frequently cited author in the *Dictionary*. The lists are evidence not only of Browne's immense erudition but his playfulness: I imagine a raised eyebrow above a twinkling eye, as he tests his readers' knowledge, and their credulity:

> *anatiferous, besprinkle, bisulcous, celestify, deoppilation, dilucidate, extispicious, exuperance, flammeous, fritinancy, guttulous, hebdomadary, illaqueation, jocundity, knabble, lixiviate, mundificative, nodosity, obtumescence, pestination, quacksalver, retromingency, solidungulous, terebrate, unridiculous, veneficial, windegg, yelk, zoographer.*

And so the author of ambiguity becomes, of course, the author of specificity. Why describe something as having two grooves in it when it can be 'bisulcous', why describe a creature as one that urinates backwards, when instead it can be praised for its 'retromingency'. It's clear that Browne delighted and luxuriated in language, and he loved to find new ways to communicate his observations with an accuracy that was in service to a necessary ambiguity.

Pseudodoxia Epidemica:

OR,

ENQUIRIES

INTO

Very many Received

TENENTS,

And commonly Presumed

TRUTHS.

By THOMAS BROWN Dr. of Physick.

The Fourth Edition.

With Marginal Observations, and a Table Alphabetical.

Whereunto are now added two Discourses

The one of URN-BURIAL, or Sepulchrall Urns, lately found in *NORFOLK*.

The other of the GARDEN of CYRUS, or Network Plantations of the Antients.

Both Newly written by the same Author.

Ex Libris colligere quæ prodiderunt Authores longe est periculosissimum Rerum ipsarum cognitio vera è rebus ipsis est. Jul. Scalig.

LONDON,

Printed for *Edward Dod*, and are to be sould by *Andrew Crook* at the *Green Dragon* in *Pauls* Church-yard.

1658.

2

CURIOSITY

a halo of wonder encircles everything that he sees ... a chamber stuffed from floor to ceiling with ivory, old iron, broken pots, urns, unicorns' horns, and magic glasses full of emerald lights and blue mystery.

Virginia Woolf
The Elizabethan Lumber Room

having seen some experiments of bitumen, and having read far more of naphtha, he whispered to my curiosity...

Religio Medici 1:19

When I first read Virginia Woolf's description of the mind and vision of Thomas Browne as encircled by a 'halo of wonder', the picture seemed to fall into my imagination fully formed, almost as if I'd read it somewhere before, or spent time picturing just such a chamber. I was at medical school then, an avid student of anatomy, and spent my summers as departmental assistant in the medical school dissecting human faces, trunks, and limbs, to facilitate the teaching of fellow students at an earlier stage of training. I wondered if Woolf's description acted as a verbal trigger of my own visual experience browsing the shelves and vitrines of Edinburgh university's anatomical museum. The collection was a rich one, gathered over four hundred years, and the items on display in the upper chambers of the building were only a fraction of what the basement held in storage. In the course of my work I sometimes had cause to descend to the basement, where catacombs of corridors extended under the fabric of the city itself, each one piled high with boxes of bones—giraffe, whale, narwhal, human—and where the shelves were loaded with body parts in formalin demonstrating the fabulous complexity and multiplicity of the animal world, as well as of the seemingly limitless possibilities of human variation.

One day at home browsing my own shelves I came upon an old copy of T.H. White's *The Sword in the Stone*, printed in 1982—the copy I had read as a child. Flicking it open near the beginning, I realized that the memory triggered by Woolf was not after all a visual one of the anatomy museum, but of a vivid act of imagination, impressed upon my childhood mind through reading White. Here is his description of the wizard Merlyn's study, which merits lengthy reproduction (even the following is abridged):

> There was a real corkindrill hanging from the rafters, very lifelike and horrible with glass eyes and scaly tail stretched out behind it. When its master came into the room it winked one eye in salutation, though it was stuffed. There were hundreds of thousands of brown books in leather bindings, some chained to the bookshelves and others propped up against each other as if they had had too much spirits to drink and did not really trust themselves. These gave out a smell of must and solid brownness which was most secure. Then there were stuffed birds, popinjays, and maggot-pies and kingfishers, and peacocks with all their feathers but two, and tiny birds like beetles, and a reputed phoenix which smelt of incense and cinnamon. It could not have been a real phoenix, because there is only one of these at a time .... There were several boars' tusks and the claws of tigers and libbards mounted in symmetrical patterns, and a big head of Ovis Poli, six live grass snakes in a kind of aquarium, some nests of the solitary wasp nicely set up in a glass cylinder, and ordinary beehive whose inhabitants went in and out

> of the window unmolested, two young hedgehogs in cotton wool, a pair of badgers which immediately began to cry Yik-Yik-Yik-Yik in loud voices as soon as the magician appeared, twenty boxes which contained stick caterpillars and sixths of the puss-moth, and even an oleander that was worth two and six, all feeding on the appropriate leaves, a guncase with all sorts of weapons which would not be invented for half a thousand years, a rob-box ditto, a lovely chest of drawers full of salmon flies which had been tied by Merlyn himself, another chest whose drawers were labelled Mandragora, Mandrake, Old Man's Beard, etc., a bunch of turkey feathers and goose-quills for making pens, an astrolabe, twelve pairs of boots, a dozen purse-nets, three dozen rabbit wires, twelve cork-screws, an ant's nest between two glass plates, ink-bottles of every possible colour from red to violet, darning needles, a gold medal for being the best scholar at Eton.[1]

That is the kind of study I'd always longed for—a vastly enlarged version of the shelves of curiosities I'd collected in my own bedroom as a child, themselves inspired by the books of Gerald Durrell, both the memoirs (e.g. *My Family and Other Animals*) and the 'how-to' books of nature that my parents bought me on birthdays (e.g. *The Amateur Naturalist*). I recognized it in a description of the rooms of the physician-naturalist Edward Wilson, the doctor who accompanied Robert Falcon Scott to the South Pole (and died with him on his return), which were 'full of skulls, flowers, birds' nests and birds' eggs'. I recognized it too in the writer Helen Macdonald's description of her own childhood bedroom:

> There were galls, feathers, seeds, pine cones, loose single wings of small tortoiseshell or peacock butterflies picked from spiders' webs, the severed wings of dead birds, spread and pinned on to cardboard to dry, the skulls of small creatures, pellets—tawny owl, barn owl, kestrel—and old bird nests.[2]

And it's there too in a frustratingly brief contemporary eyewitness account of Browne's *real* rooms, visited in October 1671 by the diarist John Evelyn:

> Next morning, I went to see Sir Thomas Browne (with whom I had some time corresponded by letter, though I had never seen him before); his whole house and garden being a paradise and cabinet of rarities; and that of the best collection, especially medals, books, plants, and natural things. Among other curiosities, Sir Thomas had a collection of the eggs of all the fowl and birds he could procure, that country (especially the promontory of Norfolk) being frequented, as he said, by several kinds which seldom or never go further into the land, as cranes, storks, eagles, and variety of water fowl. He led me to see all the remarkable places of this ancient city, being one of the largest, and certainly, after London, one of the noblest of England.[3]

And so on—into Evelyn's considerations of real estate, and the economy of England's second city. It's a frustrating account, because a fuller description of Browne's study, and home, one even half as comprehensive as White's fictional description of Merlyn's rooms, would be transformative for our understanding of Browne's attitudes of mind and in particular, of his curiosities.

He had a diligent and unflagging curiosity about *everything*, and sought to determine the truth of his enquiries by direct observation wherever possible. This is most obvious in the writings of *Vulgar Errors*, but is evident everywhere in his books. His accounts of experiments on animals might seem brutal to a modern reader, as his meditations on death might seem morbid, but I have the sense on reading him not of cruelty, but of curiosity. His contemporary Descartes viewed animals as machines, and notoriously conducted live dissections of dogs because he believed their howls of distress to be purely reflex. In Browne's less extreme view, God created animals to be in service to man, and it was appropriate to put their lives to the service of his understanding.

One of his biographers lists just a few of the practical enquiries he engaged in. He froze eggs and tested substances for their behaviour under magnetism, he fed glass and various plants to dogs to prove they were not poisonous, dissected horses, pigeons, snails, and toads, explored the transformations of tadpoles and frogs, fed cheese and bran to vipers, kept an ostrich—marvelling at how it swallowed—and fed iron to poultry to gauge the effects. His experiments were not quite the kind of thing a child might manage to conduct in the home, but almost—he didn't form hypotheses and then go out to find the animals or substances to put that hypothesis to experiment, rather he took what he had to hand. One passage in *Vulgar Errors* describes what he did when he found some deathwatch beetles. These little beetles make a ticking sound, heard within the woodwork most often in summer time—a sound which in Browne's day was widely considered a bad omen, presaging a death in the family. Rather than kill them, he 'kept them in thin boxes, wherein I have heard and seen them work and knack with a little *proboscis* or trunk against the side of the box, like a ... Woodpecker against a tree'.[4] He recommends that others do likewise, to reassure themselves and 'prevent many cold sweats in grandmothers and nurses, who in the sickness of children are so startled with these noises'. The range and cruelty of his various experiments on frogs have to be read to be believed. Curious about the ferocity of moles above ground, he placed one in a jar with a toad and a viper, and watched as it dispatched both. He wondered whether elephants fart from their trunks. His investigation of the anatomy and physiology of the sperm whale, when he encountered one beached, are justly famous:

> Out of the head of the whale, having been dead divers days, and under putrefaction, flowed streams of oil and spermaceti; which was carefully taken up and preserved by the coasters. But upon breaking up, the magazine of spermaceti, was found in the head lying in folds and courses, in the bigness of goose eggs, encompassed with large flaxy substances, as large as a mans head, in the form of honey-combs, very white and full of oil .... Had the abominable scent permitted, enquiry had been made into that strange composure of the head, and hillock of flesh about it.[5]

He wished he could have examined its throat, its bladder, the sphincter controlling its spout, and in particular had the opportunity to compare its semen with the spermaceti oil, to see what the similarities and differences might be, but couldn't get close enough—'insufferable fetor denying that enquiry'.

'The world was made to be inhabited by beasts', Browne wrote elsewhere, 'but studied and contemplated by man',[6] and it's humanity that fulfils the other element of his curiosity—in particular, himself. The grand, expansive self-affirmation of *Religio Medici* seems a precursor to Walt Whitman's poem *Song of Myself*, that freely marvels at the galaxies of wonder carried within each human frame.

> The world that I regard is myself; it is the microcosm of my own frame that I cast mine eye on; for the other, I use it but like my globe, and turn it round sometimes for my recreation. Men that look upon my outside, perusing only my condition and fortunes, do err in my altitude, for I am above Atlas's shoulders. The earth is a point, not only in respect of the heavens above us, but of that heavenly and

> celestial part within us; that mass of flesh that circumscribes me limits not my mind; that surface that tells the heaven it has an end cannot persuade me I have any. I take my circle to be above three hundred and sixty. Though the number of the arc do measure my body it comprehends not my mind. Whilst I study to find how I am a microcosm, or little world, I find myself something more than the great. There is surely a piece of divinity in us, something that was before the elements, and owes no homage unto the sun. Nature tells me I am the image of God, as well as Scripture. He that understands not thus much has not his introduction, or first lesson, and is yet to begin the alphabet of man.[7]

He cracks open the skulls of animals, and finds no convincing difference between their brains and those of man, in particular nothing that suggests itself as the seat of reason (unlike Descartes, who notoriously sited the soul in the pineal gland which, far from peculiar to humans, is a fairly primitive light-sensitive part of the brain, found in the lowest of vertebrates, which governs our bodies' sensitivity and reaction to changing day length and the seasons). That he can find nothing special in the human skull suggests to him that the soul is entirely inorganic, and leaves no material trace, and his puzzlement at the discovery inspires not irritation but wonder. His prose describing this search for the soul rolls like the sea, in a syntax of successive waves, positive followed relentlessly by negative: 'Thus we are men, and we know not how; there is something in us that can be without us, and will be after us, though it is strange that it has no history what it was before us, nor cannot tell how it entered in us.'[8]

Though he can find no imprint of the soul on the brain's anatomy, everywhere he looks within the human body seems to carry the signature of divine intervention, and perhaps this is why despite his immense learning, his relentless curiosity, Browne made little in the way of significant contributions to the then nascent disciplines of science. He is simply too busy being lost in the wonder of what he sees. Anatomizing the human body fills him with the kind of stunned sense of overwhelming glory I recognize from those summers I spent through medical school as an anatomist, preparing specimens for the teaching year, perpetually astonished by just how intricate, finely calibrated, and close-packed is the physiological machinery that keeps us alive. When in the *Garden of Cyrus* Browne considers rhomboid shapes and figures of five in nature, he takes the reader into a journey beneath the skin, where reticulations of veins, nerves, and arteries seem to him criss-crossed like those diamond patterns he has observed in plants, and his words sound like a description of the layers of abdominal muscles that overlap one another in oblique, horizontal, and reverse-oblique lines, to better buttress our vital organs: 'Thou hast curiously embroidered me', he says, claiming to extend the metaphor of human creation in scripture, 'thou hast wrought me up after the finest way of texture, and as it were with a needle.'[9]

One of Browne's publishers, Thomas Tenison, introduced the posthumous collection *Miscellany Tracts* by specifically calling upon the reader to be transported by Browne's curiosity about the world—a curiosity all the easier to follow because of his concision in writing, and wide learning: '*the Reader may content himself with these present Tracts; all which commending themselves by their Learning, Curiosity and Brevity.*' Tenison adds that anyone displeased with the contents of the book must be 'distempered' in the imagination to such a degree that he feels no obligation to respond. One of the tracts discusses the Pythian oracle, and Browne sums up his belief that our own hard work is the only oracle we should rely upon, and rather than call upon Apollo to solve our problems, we should fall upon our reason.

*

In English, the word 'curiosity' has several layers of meaning; it shares an etymology with 'care', in the sense of 'diligent' and 'eagerly enquiring'. Though I've so far considered Browne's curiosity as something to be emulated and admired, allied as it was with such a deep love of learning and a commitment to industriousness, 'curiosity' also carries the sense of something trivial and trifling, esoteric and quaint. Coleridge described Browne as someone 'Fond of the Curious, and a Hunter of Oddities & Strangenesses'. This oddity and triviality seemed to Coleridge most on display in *The Garden of Cyrus*:

> the same attention to oddities, the same to the minutenesses, & minutiae of vegetable forms—the same entireness of subject—Quincunxes in Heaven above. Quincunxes in Earth below, & Quincunxes in the water beneath the Earth; Quincunxes in Deity, Quincunxes in the mind of man; Quincunxes in bones, in optic nerves, in Roots of Trees, in leaves, in petals, in every thing![10]

Samuel Johnson thought the *Garden of Cyrus*'s companion, *Urn Burial* was the fullest expression of this tendency of Browne to lose himself in tiny details which, though arguably interesting enough, were of no real consequence—full of ultimately useless information:

> it is of small importance to know which nation buried their dead in the ground, which threw them into the sea, or which gave them to birds and beasts; when the practice of cremation began, or when it was disused; whether the bones of different persons were mingled in the same urn; what oblations were thrown into the pyre; or

> how the ashes of the body were distinguished from those of other substances.[11]

Browne's writing, from Johnson's point of view, was *just* a curiosity, nothing more. It's an observation that tells us more about Johnson and his impatient sense of urgency, his requirement for knowledge to be utilitarian, than it tells us about the value of Browne's reflections and fascinations.

*

To read Browne's attempts to satisfy his own curiosity is to get a glimpse of a pre-scientific mind at work. I love to read him because I feel as if his explorations connect my own world, my own practice of medicine, into a very particular legacy—a legacy of open-minded enquiry that is good-humoured, at ease with wonder, widely read, but also content with mystery if not with mystification. I wonder what he would have made of *Pub Med* or of *Google Scholar*, in which the world's scientific publications are listed, ranked, searchable, and where it's possible, if not to find a definitive answer to almost any scientific question one can formulate, at least to find out who has investigated your question before you, gauge how carefully their study was designed, and discern whether the results obtained reach statistical significance. This to me seems to be one of the great boons offered by the internet.

It's not in his proto-scientific enquiries into errors that I find Browne's most enthralling tussles with his emerging belief in rational enquiry, but in the pages of his book on faith, *Religio Medici*. He considers that Sodom and Gomorrah are known to have been built on ground rich in natural bitumen, and so might be expected to have become engulfed in flames through natural rather than divine means. He concedes that manna 'from heaven' is 'plentifully gathered in Calabria'[12] and has read that it was ever plentiful in Arabia—so why should it be a miracle that Moses found some? That Noah sent a pigeon from the ark that did not return he doesn't doubt, but questions why that pigeon wouldn't return for its mate, presumably still sequestered in the hold. He can trust that Lazarus was raised from the dead, but questions in what antechamber of the afterlife his soul waited for Jesus to resurrect him. 'Thus the Devil played at Chess with me', he writes of this application of the developing muscles of reason to the stories of the Bible, 'and yielding a Pawn, thought to gain a Queen of me ... whilst I laboured to raise the structure of my Reason, he strived to undermine the edifice of my Faith'.[13]

Woolf saw his mind as a kind of Wunderkammer, 'stuffed' with magic and wonder, but felt too that his focus on the human made him the precursor of novelists and autobiographers. For Herman Melville he was a 'crack'd Archangel' and if so, he's an angel preoccupied with exploring the earth and questioning the human condition. That Browne's curiosity about Lazarus, Gomorrah, Noah's Ark, and Moses' manna sits happily alongside his curiosity about toads, insects, sperm whales, and the comparative anatomy of brains, alerts me to a profoundly open intelligence, at ease with contradiction. His blurring of what are all too often set up as boundaries between disciplines of knowledge is something to be admired—knowledge is endless, and in some sense indivisible, unfiltered like the jumbled shelves of the anatomy museum or the hectic collection of Merlyn's study. When, in *The Sword in the Stone,* Merlyn announces that he will teach the boy Arthur all that he knows, the boy shouts out in a mixture of pleasure and anticipation, 'while his eyes sparkled with excitement at the discovery'.

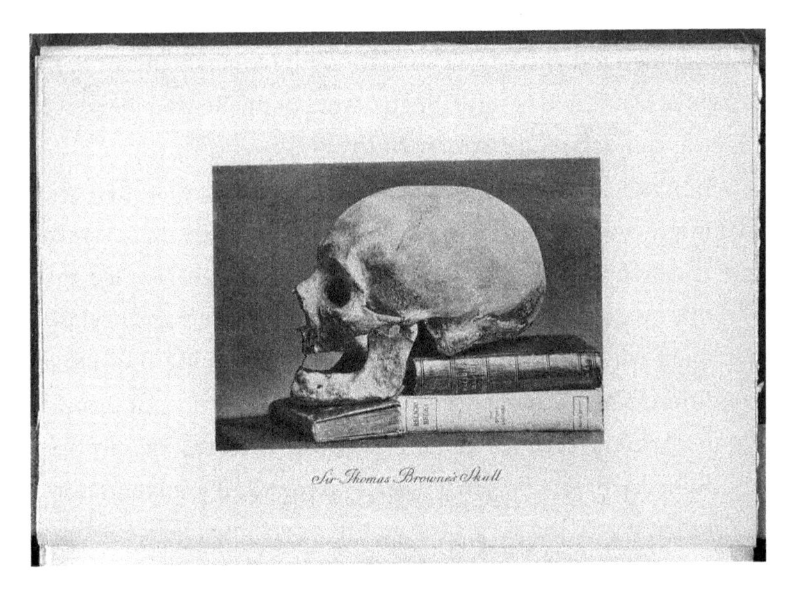

Sir Thomas Browne's Skull

3

VITALITY

metamorphosis here begins to represent vitality itself.

Marina Warner, *Fantastic Metamorphoses*

Rain water, which appearing pure and empty, is full of seminal principles, and carries vital atoms of plants and animals in it, which have not perished in the great circulation of nature.

Vulgar Errors, Of the Chameleon

Browne felt an affinity for the planet Saturn, considered harbinger of melancholy, and wrote that he was born under its sign. In his book *Religio Medici* he added that, 'I think I have a piece of that Leaden Planet in me.'[1] Browne's work has inspired many other writers over the centuries, among them the German novelist W.G. Sebald, who wrote in his *The Rings of Saturn* that 'as a doctor who saw disease growing and raging in bodies, [Browne] understood mortality better than the flowering of life.'[2] Sebald too considered himself saturnine by nature, ruled by the planet of melancholy, and the famous epigraph of his book is described as a quote from a German encyclopaedia about that planet's rings:

> The rings of Saturn consist of ice crystals and probably meteorite particles describing circular orbits around the planet's equator. In all likelihood these are fragments of a former moon that was too close to the planet and was destroyed by its tidal effect.

It's to be understood that the beauty and symmetry of Saturn's rings are the product of a cataclysmic wreck, a celestial body ripped apart by its own gravity. The birth of the rings became possible through the death of a moon. Sebald's book is an exploration of historical atrocities and injustices, whirling across the pages together with fragments from the writings of Browne, who acts not so much as a guide but as an anchor, or even as ballast. Moored by Browne's certainties, and orientated by his questing, questioning nature, Sebald arranges the broken debris of Norfolk and Suffolk's history into something new, whole, and strangely beautiful.

The idea of the unity of opposites, of birth and death, must go back to the origins of human thought, to the first hominid who realized that eating to live necessarily involves killing—what Aristotle called *allelophagia* or mutual eating. The pre-Socratic, riddling philosopher Heraclitus gave as an example the bow, which can only assume its purpose when being pulled in opposite directions. Like the bow, life exists through a tension between birth and death. Even the bow's name in Greek, '*bió̱s*' is a pun on the word for life: '*bí̱os*'. 'The bow's name is life', wrote Heraclitus, 'but its work is death.' Thomas Mann took this tension further in *The Magic Mountain*, when he described life as a 'half-sweet, half-painful balancing, or scarcely balancing, in this restricted and feverish process of decay and renewal, upon the point of existence'.[3]

As a physician, like Browne, I'm more frequently a knowing witness to death than to the creation of new life. The generation of new life in human beings is something we've only recently in our history begun to understand, and to visualize, thanks to the near miracle of IVF. But to watch IVF in action is oddly unremarkable—drips of fluid, coagulating in a petri dish. The reality within the dish, of teeming, braiding strands of DNA dancing a new being into existence, remains unseen, and was only just becoming conceivable in Browne's day.

Through reading the *Philosophical Transactions of the Royal Society*, Browne was familiar with Leeuwenhoek's revelations about the existence of spermatozoa—as he wrote to his son Edward: 'such a vast number of little animals in the melt of a cod, or the liquor which runs from it; as also in a pike; and compute that they exceed the number of men upon the whole earth at one time'.[4] Browne would have been enthralled by a modern IVF clinic; for Claire Preston, he looked at the 'miracle of germination and generation' and saw it as the 'divine signature of everlasting life'.[5]

He spent hours scrutinizing jars of pond water 'though the observation be hard', waiting for the first sign of growing duckweed to appear visible to the naked eye. He saw the emergence of new life in this way as offering insight into the very nature of creation 'wherein the leaves & root will suddenly appear where you suspected nothing before. And if the water be never so narrowly watched, yet if you can perceive any alteration of atoms as big as a needle's point, within three or four hours, the plant will be discoverable.'[6]

The transformations of death would of course have been more obvious to his human sight: within moments the skin sags, then hardens; the shifting gantries of muscle protein that in life animate our bodies begin quickly to stiffen and interlock, and will only soften again through decomposition. Blood sinks away from the uppermost skin through gravity, leaving behind the fabled 'pallor' of death. In an elaborate experiment a century ago, a Massachusetts physician called Duncan MacDougall must have watched many such extinctions: he arranged his dying patients on a scale in order to calculate the loss of weight of the soul at the very moment it departed. His calculated weight (21 grammes), was a fiction, but two and a half centuries before him, Browne already knew that the essence of vitality is no more heavy than a flame:

> [T]here may be (for ought I know) an universal and common spirit to the whole world ... However, I am sure there is a common spirit that plays within us, yet makes no part of us, and that is the spirit of God, the fire and scintillation of that noble and mighty essence, which is the life and radical heat of spirits, and those essences that know not the virtue of the Sun.[7]

For Browne, the spark of life connects us back through our ancestors to the world's creation as outlined in Genesis; the spirit that moves within us is an expression of the same dynamism with which God summoned life from the elements.

> This is that gentle heat that brooded on the waters and in six days hatched the world; this is that irradiation that dispels the mists of Hell, the clouds of horror, fear, sorrow and despair; and preserves the region of the mind in serenity: whosoever feels not the warm gale and gentle ventilation of this Spirit, (though I feel his pulse) I dare not say he lives; for truly without this, to me there is no heat under the Tropic; nor any light, though I dwelt in the body of the Sun.[8]

So Browne knew that death occasions no loss of matter. In *Vulgar Errors,* he puts his inveterate curiosity on the page when he casually debunks the common belief that dead animals weigh more than the living. He describes setting upon some scales (calibrated so finely as to 'turn upon the eighth or tenth part of a grain') some chickens and mice before death, strangling them, then reweighing them—he notices that their weight is at first the same, and then after 'eight or ten hours', begins ever so slowly to diminish.[9] He realizes that the illusion of greater heaviness in 'dead weights' is because living weights tend to help those who lift them, but the dead, being destitute of any motion 'confer no relief unto the agents, or elevators'.[10] There is then no change in gravity's hold on our bodies as they transition into death. As a process, it's simply the silencing of the intracellular clatter that sustains us, and the release of 'spirit' back to its creator—however the concept of 'spirit' or even of 'creation' is understood.

At the bedsides of patients I've often observed this transition, and transformation, as death makes its presence felt. It *does* feel as if some spiritual essence has departed, as if a soul has vacated, as if vitality itself has been dispelled. As if were we only aware of the right words to conjure, that spirit could be summoned back into what we call for good reason *mortal remains*.

*

What, then, was this vital essence for Browne? He spent much time examining the seeds of many different kinds of plants to discern the nature of the *punctilio*, or seminal element, and was amazed by how the tiniest of seeds could grow into the most enormous of trees. He wondered whether different elements of a plant had to be whole and unmutilated in order to generate a seed with the potential of growing whole, and marvelled at what was then a common misconception, that flies were generated from rotting matter of many different kinds, even from living plants (he noticed that oak trees, for example, have greater number of insects cohabiting their leaves and bark than any other tree, and believed them to be generated by the oak itself).

> The great variety of flies lies in the variety of their originals, in the seeds of caterpillars or cankers there lies not only a butterfly or moth, but if they be sterile or untimely cast, their production is often a fly ... to omit the generation of bees out of the bodies of dead heifers, or what is strange yet well attested, the production of eels in the backs of living cods and perches.[11]

He wasn't able to witness flies laying eggs, and so assumed they were generated from the rotting of matter. He wrote of how the metamorphosis of silk worms into moths was a transformation potent enough to turn his philosophy to divinity, but didn't pursue his enquiries with rigorous experiments. He knew the Greek word for butterfly is *psyche,* or 'soul', emblematic of transcendence, but didn't have the tools to observe how within its chrysalis a larva will dissolve and rebuild itself piece by piece, dying as a caterpillar before it can be reborn as a butterfly.

In his *On the Origin of Species,* Charles Darwin noted with interest how seeds carried on the sea within the crops of dead birds would often sprout, offering new life from death,* and this observation was also prefigured in Browne's meditations on the subject: 'Seeds found in wildfowls gizards have sprouted in the earth.'[12] But it's Browne's meditations on mammalian reproduction that offer a fascinating insight into an intelligence deeply read in the classical texts of sex and heredity, and illustrate how much the views he held were alive and influential well into the nineteenth century.

Pythagoras was one of the earliest philosophers of heredity when he suggested that each man's semen was a distillate of his physical attributes—a position later called 'spermism'. Predominant classical belief was that female genitalia was an

* 'the carcasses of birds, when floating on the sea, sometimes escape being immediately devoured; and seeds of many kinds in the crops of floating birds long retain their vitality'.

arrested version of the male, and the role of women in conception and embryogenesis was that of soil, rather than seed. Aristotle conceded a greater role for women but still thought there was no specific female generative seed, something Browne discusses in detail in *Vulgar Errors*, when he considers a story he'd read in Averroes—which reports on a woman who conceived without sexual intercourse after sharing a bath with a man.

> The relation of Averroes, and now common in every mouth, of the woman that conceived in a bath, by attracting the sperm or seminal effluxion of a man admitted to bath in some vicinity unto her, I have scarce faith to believe; and had I been of the jury, should have hardly thought I had found the father in the person that stood by her. 'Tis a new and unseconded way in history to fornicate at a distance, and much offends the rules of physic, which say, there is no generation without a joint emission, nor only a virtual, but corporal and carnal contact. And although Aristotle and his adherents do cut off the one, who conceive no effectual ejaculation in women, yet in defence of the other they cannot be introduced ... And therefore that conceit concerning the daughters of Lot, that they were impregnated by their sleeping father, or conceived by seminal pollution received at distance from him, will hardly be admitted.[13]

Aristotle did add the insight that new human beings were created not through the transformation of semen *per se*, but through instructions carried in the semen: '[Just as] no material part comes from the carpenter to the wood in which he works, but the shape and the form are imparted from him to the material by means of the motion he sets up ... In like manner, Nature uses the semen as a tool.'[14] The Nobel laureate and biophysicist Max Delbrück suggested that with this observation, Aristotle foresaw the existence of DNA, and should perhaps be awarded a posthumous Nobel Prize.

Variants of Pythagorean spermism persisted, with attendant misogyny: the earliest microscopists saw tiny homunculi curled in the heads of spermatozoa, and in the seventeenth century the Dutch biologist Jan Swammerdam could assert 'in Nature there is no generation, but only propagation, the growth of parts. Thus original sin is explained, for all men were contained in the organs of Adam and Eve. When their stock of eggs is finished, the human race will cease to be.'[15] Within their gonads, homunculi carried within them other homunculi *ad infinitum*, all the way back to Adam, giving natural philosophers steeped in Calvinist theology a biological explanation for the persistence of original sin. Browne suggested Adam's ribs contained seminal elements, otherwise Eve could not have been created from them: 'although her production were not by copulation, yet was it in a manner seminal.'[16]

Even Charles Darwin's earliest theories of heredity entertained a variant of Pythagorean spermism—Darwin suggested that hereditary units called 'gemmules' absorbed elements of each parent's characteristics, and these gemmules were then concentrated in the gonads. The process wasn't perfect, and variations crept in, giving rise to what he called 'sports' and would later be called 'mutants' (Darwin's theory of the origin of species by natural selection didn't require an intimate knowledge of the mechanism of heredity, only an observation of its effects).

It's startling that Pythagorean and Aristotelian notions of heredity persisted into the Victorian period, and that we have advanced in just 150 years to the frankly astonishing position where we can now edit the genes of embryos and target therapies specific to an individual's DNA. Aristotle thought of this germinative element in life as a set of instructions for a kind of motion capable of transforming elements into certain patterns. He'd have had no way, of course, of understanding DNA as a particular type of molecule, or that it's a molecule that has the ability to generate proteins, or that proteins through their actions render matter capable of supporting life.

Browne saw that this depth of analysis was beyond him, beyond even the reach of Swammerdam's microscopes: 'The forms of things may lie deeper then we conceive them; seminal principles may not be dead in the divided atoms of plants: but wandering in the ocean of nature, when they hit upon proportionable materials, may unite, and return to their visible selves again.'[17] This seems to me a beautiful summary of the elemental recycling of lifegiving elements, all that carbon, hydrogen, nitrogen, and phosphorus, that constitutes our own bodies even as it composed the bodies of dinosaurs, of trilobites, and those primitive cyanobacteria that first colonized the seas.

*

A biochemist called Aleksandr Oparin introduced the idea of life's origin from 'primordial soup' at a meeting of the Russian Biochemical Society in 1922. Oparin suggested that the Earth's seas once foamed with a broth of amino acids and simple fats that combined to create the first simple organisms. He showed that amino acids have the power to self-organize into protein chains, and that biochemical processes work better when encased in droplets of gelatin and gum—substances he used to make primitive cell walls. His theory was written up and published in 1936, under the title 'Origin of Life on Earth'.

A decade or so later two chemists called Stanley Miller and Harold Urey tested Oparin's idea. If the chemicals necessary for the generation of life had to be available in the clays and rainwaters of the early Earth, then it should be possible to generate them by recreating the Earth's initial conditions. With laboratory apparatus not unlike that in the IVF clinic, Miller made a closed tube of glass with two flasks within it and attached a condenser. He arranged the atmosphere within this closed system according to the best available theories on the atmosphere of the early Earth. One flask, containing half a pint of water, was heated and its boiling vapour passed through the second flask, where electric sparks discharged between electrodes to simulate lightning. The gaseous mixture was then cooled through the condenser, and the resulting liquid funneled back to the original flask. Miller had recreated a primordial water cycle with seas, storms, and rain clouds, and he allowed this mixture to cycle through the flasks for a week.

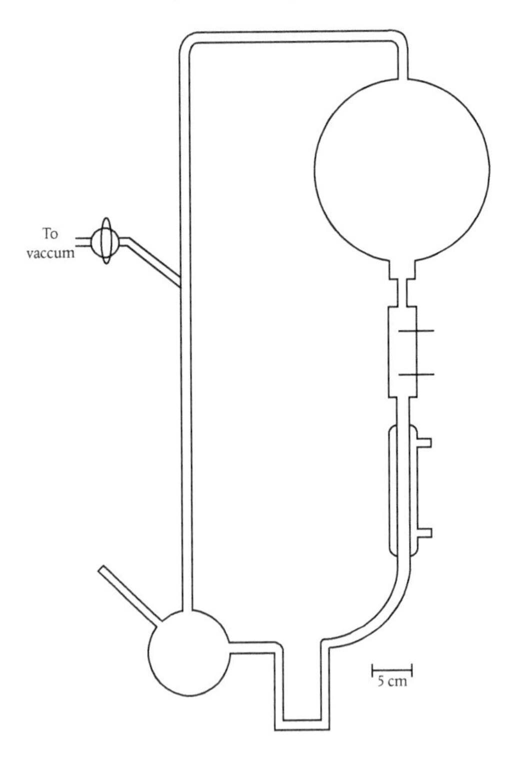

After the first day, the 'water in the flask became noticeably pink.' After a week, it became 'deep red and turbid' with newly created organic compounds. He analysed the contents of the solution: there were enough amino acids to build simple proteins.[18]

Subsequent modifications to the experimental conditions added iron compounds, silicates, and reproduced the chemical environment thought to pertain around early volcanoes. These experiments proved capable of generating scores more amino acids that could make ever more complex proteins, as well as nucleotides—the building blocks of DNA.

When I first read of Miller and Urey's experiments to create the building blocks of life, my image of their laboratory—bubbling glass flasks strobed with discharges of lightning—was inflected by movie-renditions of the laboratory of Dr Frankenstein. Mary Shelley's novel was subtitled 'The Modern Prometheus', because its hero, Victor Frankenstein, is both gifted and cursed by his ability to create life, just as Prometheus was blessed with great knowledge, then cursed for sharing it with the human race. 'And the moon gazed on my midnight labours', wrote Shelley of Frankenstein's laboratory, 'while, with unrelaxed and breathless eagerness, I pursued nature to her hiding-places'.[19] Dr Frankenstein is portrayed as unhinged in his crazed pursuit; by comparison Dr Browne's even-minded sanity is refreshing to read: that the 'form of things' might lie deeper than can be conceived by man is simply noted, not deplored.

Mary Shelley was one for whom the power to reanimate the dead would have been particularly welcome—her mother had died within days of her birth, and by the time she wrote *Frankenstein*, at just eighteen, had already endured the death of a baby daughter. She wrote in her diary after the latter: 'Dream that my little baby came to life again; that it had only been cold, and that we rubbed it before the fire, and it lived.' She had read the works of John Aldini, who in 1803, in London, tried to reanimate an executed criminal's body with electricity[†]—he succeeded in making the arms and facial muscles of the dead man twitch. Despite her bitter experience, and dreams of reanimation, Shelley was clear-sighted enough to imagine that the power to grant life would pose immense danger to anyone unfortunate enough to possess it. Dr Frankenstein 'desired to learn the secrets of heaven and earth ... banish disease from the human frame, and render man invulnerable to any but a violent death'.[20] But the result of his creation is quite the opposite: 'I am a blasted tree', Frankenstein says towards the end of the book, 'a miserable spectacle of wrecked humanity, pitiable to others, and intolerable to myself.'[21]

*

Sebald's *The Rings of Saturn* opens with its author having suffered in some unspoken way, broken in body and mind, looking out through a hospital window at the heavens. In one evocative, melancholy passage, he describes himself looking out east over the North Sea, filled with an awareness of the Earth's ceaseless cycles of rotation, of life and death, of the planet turning between light and darkness as if a black veil were being drawn back and forth with every nightfall. To imagine the scene from space, he falls back on Browne's metaphor from the *Garden of Cyrus*, when he describes Saturn, god of Time, wielding the sickle of death.

If there's life elsewhere in our solar system, it might well be in orbit around Saturn. The sixty or so moons of Saturn, one or more

[†] 'electricity' was one of the many words Browne had coined over a century earlier, though Aldini called the phenomenon 'Galvinism'.

of which must once have disintegrated to yield its rings, have a variety of forms and compositions. Titan is more than 5,000 kms across—bigger than Mars—and has deep-freeze subterranean oceans, as well as being the only celestial body in our solar system, other than our planet, to have surface lakes (though they are of hydrocarbons, not water). Two of Saturn's moons, Janus and Epimethus, follow orbits separated by just forty or so kilometres; every four years they meet and swap places, pirouetting past one another like dancers in a reel, or racehorses changing lanes. But it's another moon, Enceladus, that has enough melted water in it to convince astrobiologists it could harbour life. Enceladus is a white ball of ice with a magma heated core, and geyser-plumes of water from its southern pole condense to create one of Saturn's paler rings. When the space probe *Cassini* skimmed close enough to Enceladus to look for evidence of life, its instruments were grazed by those plumes, and it was almost knocked off course. The chemical constituents of Enceladus appear to be similar to those sparked and boiled in the laboratory of Miller and Urey.

The space probe Cassini was designed to fail; on 15 September 2017 it fell into the atmosphere of Saturn and incinerated. There was a concern that despite its twenty year mission across the solar system, some microorganisms, amino acids, or nucleotides might have persisted on its surface, and its designers were anxious that those biochemical imprints of life would never contaminate the planet, or any of its moons. As it tumbled with increasing speed between the innermost rings of Saturn and its upper atmosphere, powerful antennae on Earth turned towards the spacecraft to pick up on its last, dying emissions. It mapped Saturn's gravity and told astronomers just how fast the planet spins. It assessed the mass of material in Saturn's rings, and sampled the ice that had sprayed from Enceladus' core, where even now, some kindred forms of life might be in evolution. In a few billion years, when the sun becomes a red giant, it will swell to consume the Earth. By then, the only life remaining in our solar system could be in orbit around Saturn.

It's a distinction unacknowledged among the many fruits of Browne's imagination that it might one day be possible for the churning elements of life to exit Earth's gravity and drop out of circulation, neither buried nor burned on its surface, but propelled into orbit. Every living thing so far ejected from our atmosphere (among them the many dogs, monkeys, mice, tortoises, spiders, and mealworms that have so far been shot into space) has returned to Earth. Some returned as their spacecraft burned up in the atmosphere, their ashes scattering in a fine powder across the upper reaches of the sky—joining the estimated one million tons of space dust that settles daily on the Earth. But for the first time since life on Earth began, the elements of which we are composed have the potential to begin new cycles of incorporation and dissolution elsewhere in the universe. Browne would have marvelled at the idea that, from the moment the first experimental animal strikes out from Earth's orbit towards Mars, our planet will be leaking that elemental stuff of life: carbon, nitrogen, and phosphorus will exit the close circuit of the elements here to take part in a broader, more universal circuit.

*

Browne's contemporary in France, Cyrano de Bergerac (1619–1655) imagined a journey into space, to the moon, and from that lunar perspective mused on the animating principle that can forge life from dust and ashes: 'A hundred million times matter, on the way to human shape, has been stopped to form now a stone, now lead, now coral, now a flower, now a comet, and all because of more or fewer elements that were or were not necessary for designing a man.'[22] This vision of a great hierarchy of being, with god and the angels at the top, and humanity just a rung below, calls to mind Dante's spiralling journey from the inferno into paradise. It's a pattern Browne explicitly brings out in many of his writings: there is a hierarchy of being that begins in simple matter, and ascends through plants, animals, mankind, ultimately to reach its zenith in a realm of spirits and of angels. His naturalist's vision reminds me of Edward Wilson, another physician of faith, who wrote to his wife: 'Love everything into which God has put life: and God made nothing dead. There is only *less* life in a stone than in a bird, and both have a life of their own, and both took their life from God.'[23]

For Browne, we can only ever form a link in that great chain of being, stone to spirit, not its terminus, because life's fundamental underlying principles will continue forever after we are gone. 'Life is a pure flame', he wrote in *Urn Burial*, 'and we live by an invisible sun within us.'[24] In his earlier work *Religio Medici*, he took this further, staking a claim for humanity's privilege and responsibility in exemplifying the fusion of matter and spirit. Our embryological development from the moment of conception recapitulates that same hierarchy, and if we live our lives well, we can become the embodiment of a moral and ethical animal, the apogee of the development of life.

> [W]e are only that amphibious piece between a corporal and spiritual essence, that middle frame that links those two together, and makes good the method of God and nature, that jumps not from extremes, but unites the incompatible distances by some middle

> and participating natures; that we are the breath and similitude of God, it is indisputable, and upon record of holy Scripture; but to call our selves a Microcosm, or little world, I thought it only a pleasant trope of rhetoric, till my nearer judgement and second thoughts told me there was a real truth therein.[25]

It's as if Browne is consciously laying the seventeenth-century foundation to the eighteenth-century idea that in our embryological development we human beings experience all of the developmental changes of the great chain of being, a belief summarized as 'ontogeny recapitulates phylogeny'. It was a theory touched on with my own medical training in embryology, though only to mention it had been subsequently disproven. But in Browne's rendering, it's possible to see nonetheless its great metaphorical power.

> First we are a rude mass, and in the rank of creatures, which only are, and have a dull kind of being, not yet privileged with, or preferred to sense or reason; next we live the life of plants, the life of animals, the life of men, and at last the life of spirits, running on in one mysterious nature those five kinds of existences, which comprehend the creatures not of the world, only, but of the Universe.[26]

Browne's *Religio Medici* is woven through with paradox; it professes an obstinacy of faith even as it valorizes scepticism: life is seen as a great mystery, and death more mysterious still. Yet Browne sought deeper understanding of those mysteries even as he acknowledged that some questions can never be answered. Like Italo Calvino, he seems to have thought of himself as 'a Saturn who dreams of being a Mercury'.[27] Browne was candid about his own contradictions;

in a discussion of life and death he quoted Dante's antisyzygy in *the Divine Comedy*: 'I love to doubt, as well as to know.'[‡] An understanding of how vitality comes to animate matter eluded him just as it eludes us. But in his search for an answer he illuminated many mysteries, while simultaneously deepening his faith.

‡ *Inferno*, xi. 93 *'Che non men, che saver, dubbiar m'aggrata'.*

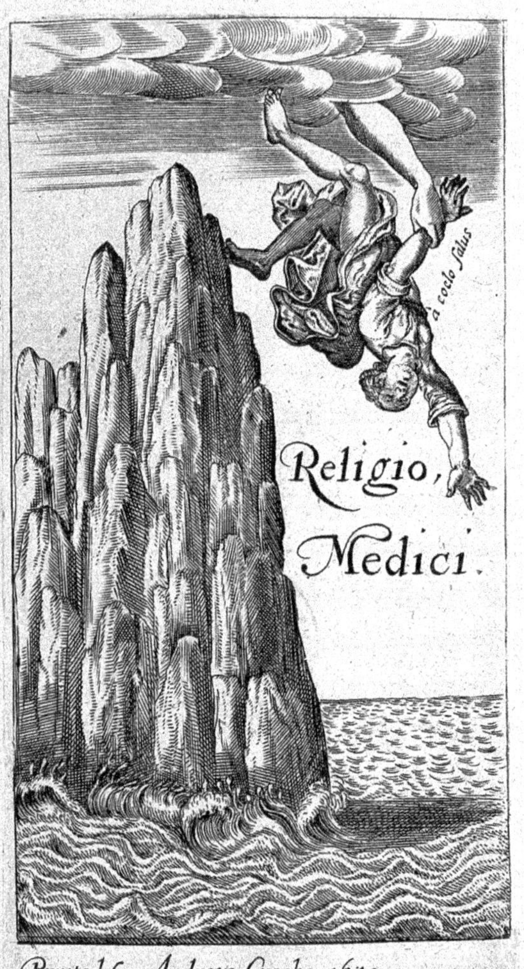
à coelo salus
Religio, Medici.
Printed for Andrew Crooke. 1642. Will: Marshall scu:

4

PIETY

I do not think that my remarks about religion made much impression upon Queequeg … he no doubt thought he knew a good deal more about the true religion than I did.

Herman Melville, *Moby Dick*

One day lived after the perfect rule of piety, is to be preferred before sinning immortality.

Letter to a Friend

The Waagebouw in Amsterdam where Rembrandt painted his famous *Anatomy Lesson of Dr Tulp* is a restaurant now rather than a weigh-house, or a guild hall for surgeons. Apparently, it has also served time as a fire station and as a museum. There were no tables free for dinner, but I ordered a beer and sat at one of the tables outside, took out my notebook, and thought about whether Thomas Browne might really have been upstairs that day with Rembrandt and Dr Tulp, as W.G. Sebald suggested in *The Rings of Saturn*. Sebald presumes Browne to have been resident in Leiden at the time, January 1632, but it's likely that Browne was still in Montpellier, en route to Italy. '[I]t is probable that Browne would have heard of the dissection and was present at the extraordinary event', Sebald nevertheless wrote, 'which Rembrandt depicted in his painting of the Guild of Surgeons, for the anatomy lessons given every year in the depth of winter by Dr Nicolaas Tulp were not only of the greatest interest to a student of medicine but constituted in addition a significant date in the agenda of a society that saw itself as emerging from the darkness into the light.' As if to underscore the auspicious nature of the occasion, Sebald suggests that in all likelihood Descartes was there too.

To reach the Waagebouw I'd walked down a lane of shop windows like the glass cases of a museum, but behind each was a naked woman beckoning to me. Ahead in the lane was a gang of jumpy Spanish teenagers, agape, serious-faced at their impiety, as if feeling themselves observed by their village priest or their mothers. Earlier that day I'd checked in to a nearby apartment with my wife and young children, and the landlady had said, 'if your children ask questions about the women in the windows, just tell them they're getting ready to go swimming in the canal.' It was November, and I was in Amsterdam to promote the Dutch translation of one of my books. At lunch with my publisher, I'd heard that the red light district's circus of gawping and vomiting tourists was beginning to test the famous toleration of the Dutch. New laws were being introduced to curb the area's attractiveness to tourism, drug users, and prostitution.

As we left the restaurant, my publisher grabbed my shoulder, pulling me back from the road and saving me from a collision. 'Watch out for the bicycles', he shouted as an oblivious cyclist whistled past, texting as she pedalled. 'If the cyclist is smiling, it's a tourist', he said; 'if frowning, they are Dutch.' But on my walks in the city that toleration for which the Netherlands are justly renowned seemed very much alive; I didn't sense much in the way of grudge or bad temper.

If it wasn't for the intervening English Channel as it opens out into the North Sea, the Netherlands and the Fens of East Anglia would be contiguous. They were even connected until a few thousand years ago by the land bridge now known as Doggerland—only a river crossing or two would have interrupted a pedestrian walking from Amsterdam to Norwich. There are similarities too in matters of religion, and in attitude to education. In the 1640s, England and the Netherlands had the highest literacy levels to be found anywhere on Earth. Studies are bedevilled by the difficulty of knowing whether someone who could sign their name was also capable of reading and writing, but it has been estimated that upwards of 30 per cent of the population were literate (most of these were men).

*

Exiting Leiden train station, the traveller is confronted by a new, modern building of beige and blue, glass and silver, with 'Leids Universitait Medisch Centrum' over its revolving doors in giant, illuminated letters—'Leiden University Medical Centre.' Inside there is a broad piazza of an entrance lobby, a little mosque behind the café, gleaming corridors and, the day I visited, tastefully arranged artworks, the strangest being a fat brown blob of a sculpture with human arms and a manatee's head, and the most interesting being a photograph of a wooden river-pier in Papua New Guinea, crowded with locals watching the photographer with expressions of amazement mingled with scorn. There was a colossal installation, the height of four storeys, in the form of an eye that had been injured—the lower parts of the chamber between pupil and cornea were filling with blood.

Leiden's medical university is still at the forefront of European medical research and of teaching. There is an exchange programme with my own university that I would have been glad to pursue as a student, but it wasn't available for my chosen subject of neuroscience. My plan to set up some meetings there had also fallen through, so after a brief exploratory tour of the hospital I left its glass and steel behind, found an underpass to get past the railway line, and walked into the Leiden that more closely approximated the one Browne would have known.

There are many canals there, cobbles of fired earth rather than stone, more bicycles, university buildings old and new, cannons, poems on the walls in their original languages—Bashō, Shakespeare—and on one splendidly decorated wall, a commemoration of the local astronomer Jan Oort, who gave his name to the conjectured spherical shell of ice and rubble, thought to encase our solar system at such an immense radius from our sun that photons take the best part of a month to reach it. Leiden struck me as a town of books, its university district centred on a library that resembled a vast, sprawling artificial heart of valves, chambers, and exposed tubular supports. I walked in the same botanical gardens that Browne knew, laid out in 1590 (fifty years after Padua, and twenty years after Bologna). On almost every street there were churches, built as they were in my own country by the irresistible pressure of Christian piety as it flowed through the continent like a glaciation. Each now appeared stranded, abandoned like so much moraine following that piety's retreat.

Browne went on to Leiden after his time as a student in Padua; his biographer Reid Barbour thought it likely that he would have reached the town via Paris. He likely had to quarantine along the way because of outbreaks of plague among the communities he passed through (plague had devastated Padua university not long before Browne's arrival, with many of the professors killed by it). It's not known how long he spent in the city, and it's probable that he was there for several months before his recorded matriculation date of 3 December 1633, attending lectures and learning the language. Matriculation was a paperwork formality, necessary before applying to be examined for an MD degree. Barbour says that he was examined by Adolph Vorstius, another graduate of Padua and chief botanist of the medical school. He lodged with one Richard Monck on the Sonneveltsteeg.

Leiden was then a town of literacy, learning, and of faith, where Browne learned the modest style of dress that he adopted ever after ('In his habit of clothing he had an aversion to all finery, and affected plainness both in fashion and ornaments.'[1]) and which influenced the pragmatic Christianity that is so much on show in *Religio Medici*. The title of that book—the Religion of a Doctor—was intended as a kind of provocation: physicians were considered the most irreligious of all professionals, their faith often questioned. '[T]hough in point of devotion & piety physicians do meet with common obloquy', Browne wrote, 'yet in the Roman Calendar we find no less then twenty-nine saints and martyrs of that profession.'[2] The comparison is disingenuous—the piety of physicians in the early days of the founding of the Christian Church can hardly be used as evidence of the same degree of religious observance in a world where society was, as Sebald observed, emerging from what was characterized as a dark degree of ignorance, into the light of deeper knowledge.

Browne thought religious relics a fraud, but balked at questioning scriptural authority when it came to matters such as the Hebrew account of Creation. It would take a further two centuries before observant thinkers could discard scripture entirely when faced with evidence such as fossil remains of sea creatures found high in the mountains. (Browne, like many others, took recourse to explanations involving the Flood.) Before James

Hutton and Charles Lyell wrote on the subject, there was no lack of evidence for the age of the Earth—it was just that the observers' rigid adherence to pious and received ideas of truth made them discard it.

His attitude to faith was a curious mixture of rigidity and flexibility, of orthodox and unorthodox. Alexander Whyte, the Scottish preacher who published a lengthy oration on the subject of *Religio Medici*, repeated a comment given by a friend that Browne's popularity in Continental Europe was because he was a 'Pelagian'—someone who didn't really believe in Original Sin, but instead held to the idea of human perfectibility on Earth. There are numerous interpretations of 'pious', after all.

Browne believed in the importance of a physician's diagnostic and therapeutic skill, but at the same time of the imperative that faith be called on to aid the healing process. He maintained that it was crucial 'to pray daily and particularly for sick patients, & in general for others, wheresoever, howsoever, under whose care soever'.[3] Before entering the homes of his patients (most of his medical encounters would have been what we now call 'home visits') he would recite 'the peace and mercy of God be in this place.' 'I cannot go to cure the body of my patient', he wrote, 'but I forget my profession and call unto God for his soul.' On his rounds, he said, he felt the obligation or desire to pray ceaselessly, like the mendicant pilgrims of the Orthodox Christian tradition, or the Hindu divines who aimed to pronounce the name of God with each breath: 'To pray in all places where privacy invites: in any house, highway, or street: and to know no street or passage in this city which may not witness that I have not forgot God and my Saviour in it.' Yet he admitted freely to doubt: 'There is, as in Philosophy, so in Divinity, sturdy doubts, and boisterous objections, wherewith the unhappiness of our knowledge too nearly acquaints us' he wrote in *Religio Medici*. Of his questions: 'more of these no man hath known than myself.'[4]

When Samuel Taylor Coleridge marked up a copy of *Religio Medici*, he wrote apropos of this passage: 'This is exceedingly striking! Had Sir T. Brown lived now-a-days, he would probably have been a very ingenious & bold Infidel (in his *real* opinions) tho' the kindness of his nature would have kept him aloof from vulgar prating obstrusive Infidelity.'[5] Coleridge didn't grapple with the implications of Browne's attitude to theology, but was simply attracted to the prose in which Browne articulated his meditations, and the way Browne was drawn to the most awkward implications of faith. For Coleridge, from his vantage point of the 1800s, Browne's piety seemed only skin deep, a gloss painted over him by the century in which he lived, and expressed in print only for the sake of appearances.

But to conceive of Browne's faith in nineteenth century terms is anachronistic, and it might be truer to his memory to take his acceptance of faith's mysteries at his word:

> As for those wingy mysteries in divinity, and airy subtleties in religion, which have unhinged the brains of better heads, they never stretched the pia mater* of mine. Methinks there be not impossibilities enough in religion for an active faith; the deepest mysteries ours contains, have not only been illustrated, but maintained by syllogism, and the rule of reason.[6]

*

'Piety' makes an appearance only once in the King James Bible. It's in Paul's first letter to Timothy (now almost universally

* The thin lining of the brain's surface.

recognized as not written by Paul). King James's translators rendered 5:4 as 'But if any widow have children or nephews, let them learn first to shew piety at home, and to requite their parents: for that is good and acceptable before God.' The Greek word used was εὐσεβεῖν—*eusebein* which can mean piety but also loyalty, respect for tradition and for your parents—something more akin to what we'd now think of as Confucian virtues than Christian ones. I asked a classicist friend what the Greek original would have meant, and she told me that literally it would be, 'let them first learn to reverence their own household', a word used by Euripides in his play *Alcestis,* in Plato's *Symposium,* and by Aeschylus in *Agamemnon,* about the reverence and respect owed to the gods. She also pointed out that the Vulgate Latin translation of the Bible, the word εὐσεβεῖν is rendered 'regere', as in '*discant primum domum suam regere*'—those widows with children and nephews were being implored to *regere* their own homes: 'lead straight', 'manage', 'govern', or 'set straight'. A concept quite far from modern understandings of 'piety'.

For this, and for other inflexions found across the writings of Browne, I suspect that our modern interpretation of piety is too narrow, buckled too tightly to a Victorian religiosity, and thus diminished in terms of its possibilities compared to the essence it held in Browne's day. What manifested as his piety was more than simply faith, but was an expression of that deep commitment to the religious tradition into which he was born, and which anchored the ship of his free-ranging mind. His insistence that 'one day lived after the perfect rule of piety, is to be preferred before sinning immortality',[7] is given a different complexion when the depths of meaning in that word, as he understood it, are explored.

Piety doesn't come into the list of traditional Christian virtues (chastity, temperance, charity, diligence, patience, kindness, and humility), though it might be thought of as influencing the way all seven of them are understood. Greek ideas of virtue condensed instead around justice, courage, and temperance, while the Hebrew Ten Commandments considered piety worth celebrating for its own sake (along with fidelity, and keeping the peace). I prefer to think that, with regard to piety, Browne would have agreed with Aristotle that for a virtue to remain virtuous, it had to be shown not in its fullest or most extreme form, but instead 'to the right person, to the right extent, at the right time'. Christian piety for its own sake was without value, and whether honouring the homes of the sick with a blessing before entering, or recalling each one of his patients in his prayers, he was in truth making a 'windmill upon a mount of dead men's bones',[8] i.e. transforming something old and dead into something of profound use to him for his life and his work.

In modern medical practice it's a brave or foolish doctor that would invoke piety or faith to assist the recovery of his or her patients. In their conception of health, modern medical practitioners like myself are more likely to invoke humanity's ceaseless bombardment by viruses, the complexities of our inadequately understood nutrition, the effect of neurotransmitters on mood, or the still uncharted dynamic between our microbiome and our immune systems. But in many ways we're no different from Browne, who also took advantage of his own time's prevailing currents of thought to explain illness in ways that his patients could make sense of. Health, too, is a balance between extremes, not an extreme in itself, and in my own consultations I try to find out what my patient has most faith in, before formulating a plan that might help them to recover health. Drugs and therapies are only a small part of healing—much of how we get better is determined by our expectations, and by our beliefs.

Through modern scientific trials we know that someone's faith in a particular cure profoundly influences its effectiveness. Placebo drugs are a good example of this, and study after study has proven how useful they can be as treatments. Capsule formulations of medication are perceived as more effective than tablets; red and yellow pills make better stimulants, while blue and green make better sedatives. Scientific knowledge is a necessary foundation to Western medical practice but is sadly insufficient on its own; to be effective, a physician often has to reach into his or her patients' belief system and prescribe a treatment that will make sense in context. When faced with someone who has an unshakeable faith in medication but a condition that responds poorly to drugs, I often wish I had access to the kind of placebos that made up much of Browne's pharmacopoeia. It's the least that my patients expect—and expectations make powerful remedies.

*

Western European piety as Browne understood it is largely in retreat. Roman Catholicism has experienced a bombardment of corruption and sex scandals across the clergy, from village priests to the high officials of the Vatican. Protestant traditions continue to splinter into a myriad of sects, and the Church in which I grew up, the Church of Scotland, has lost half of its adherents in just the last twenty years. The glittering successes of the scientific method have led many to put their faith in science, not God, and with the development of welfare states, churches have lost their role as the principal providers of charity.

My own upbringing was within a small village community divided between the Church of Scotland I attended, and a nearby Roman Catholic church; I remember at the age of three or four my astonishment at learning my Catholic friends would attend a separate school from my own. I wanted to know immediately why it was that Catholics didn't then have a separate swimming pool too. For young children, the endless divisions promoted by faiths make no sense; as I get older I feel as if I'm returning to that position.

The former Anglican Bishop of Edinburgh, Richard Holloway, told me once that he now thinks of religion as an art form, one of humanity's most creative, dedicated across millennia to answering the great puzzles of human life: What are we doing here? What happens after death? Why is there suffering? How should we live? It offers consolation, moral guidance, and reassurance, even as it fosters guilt and division. His words made me think of a lecture I heard once by the Dalai Lama, when I was working as a doctor in a small hospital that served the Tibetan refugees in India. He began by counselling young Westerners (who hung on his every word) to stick to their own religious traditions rather than adopt Buddhism. Each faith was only a door after all, opening into a state that must by necessity be universally accessible to all human beings. From this point of view, his brand of Buddhism was no better or worse than any of the other world faiths. All were comparable when practised with compassion and genuine humility, rather than with slavish adherence to obsolete texts. All had the potential to offer answers to those great puzzles of human existence.

Browne loved paradox, and though he proclaimed that he would like to see Anglicanism spread over the globe, his writings themselves betray an ease with alternative interpretations of scripture, and show respect for different religious persuasions. The traditions embedded in the thinking with which I approach the great puzzles of human existence have their roots in Christian Europe, but have been overlain in the centuries since Browne with new modes of enquiry—of science and philosophy—and new revelations not just of the complexity of the natural world but of the possibilities of human societies. If we take piety in its old sense as respect for tradition, then to be pious isn't perhaps such a bad idea, and is even compatible with innovation and faith in the future. As Europeans we've yet to take the best from our own traditions, and many possibilities for how to build on them remain unexplored.

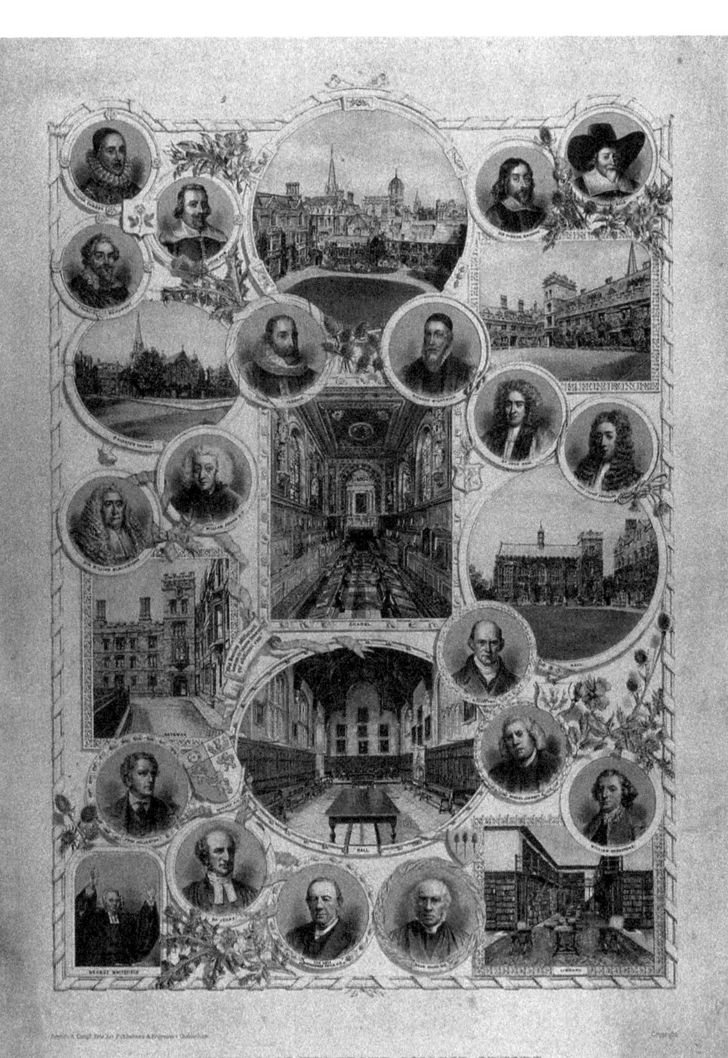

MEMORIAL OF PEMBROKE COLLEGE, OXFORD.

5

HUMILITY

All streams flow to the sea because it is lower than they are. Humility gives it its power.

Tao Te Ching, 66

we are not magisterial in opinions, nor have we dictator-like obtruded our conceptions; but in the humility of enquiries or disquisitions, have only proposed them unto more ocular discerners...

Vulgar Errors, Introduction

It's unusual for physicians to admit to a lack of knowledge, to doubt, or to volunteer that sometimes decades of research and study can leave us with more questions than we started out with. It's as if faced the with the pressure to cure, some of my colleagues are afraid of exposing their own vulnerabilities and uncertainties, and prefer to hold up a kind of rigid mask of professional competence with which they hope to save face. My own medical practice is saved from the worst of this kind of bluffing because of its generalism: no one expects a general practitioner to be knowledgeable about the details of everything.* The word *humility* itself is out of fashion today, given how much our own age values self-confidence and self-affirmation, but to discover something new, it's necessary first to acknowledge the limits of one's own understanding.

One of Browne's admirable qualities was his capacity to admit to uncertainty, and his lengthiest work, *Vulgar Errors*, was itself

* The breadth of knowledge GPs are expected to be conversant in can still be formidable: I have been asked by a patient if I can fix their boiler.

a systematic examination of the limits of knowledge and an exploration, often by trial and error, of received wisdoms. This was at the inception of the scientific revolution and the new natural philosophers were seeking to challenge *everything*, to sweep aside centuries of folk assumptions about the way the world works, and start anew.

I admire Browne's openness to being wrong, recognizing in him the humility of the non-specialist. Those who knew him remarked upon it as something unexpected in a man so well-travelled and well-read. One acquaintance, Reverend John Whitefoot of Heigham in Norfolk, wrote in his *Minutes for the Life of Sir Thomas Browne*, 'His modesty was visible in a natural habitual blush, which was increased upon the least occasion, and oft discovered without any observable cause. Those who knew him only by the briskness of his writings were astonished at his gravity of aspect and countenance, and freedom from loquacity.'[1]

He was in correspondence with some of the greatest minds of his day, but Browne was never a member of the Royal Society, and today his only real contributions to knowledge are considered the first description of *adipocere*, or 'grave-wax' (the oily concretion left in the soil following the long dissolution of interred bodies) and an observation regarding electricity. That his contributions to science have ultimately proven to be modest is perhaps appropriate for a man so guided by the virtue of humility. Though he considered *Vulgar Errors* his masterpiece, he is remembered far more now for his authorship of *Religio Medici*, as a searching examination of his Anglican faith and how it was in accord or discord with his profession of medicine. He was embarrassed, in later years, by some of the immaturities on display in the work, but is remembered today far more as its author than he is remembered as a doctor.

Despite the 1,400 pages of his works in my edition,[2] it's clear that Browne had further unexplored ideas, sufficient to fill a whole library of books. We must content ourselves with fragments of these, and seek value in what was left unfinished. The demands of family and of professional life must have been an obstacle to his committing many of his ideas to paper. At the same time I have the sense on reading him that family life was for him not an irritation or an obstacle, but instead an obligatory part of all life: to give back, from gratitude, more into the life that created him.

For physician-writers the profession of medicine is the means by which they are granted both liberation from the need to earn money from writing (Samuel Johnson: 'No man but a blockhead ever wrote, except for money'), and inspiration for what they write. They're fortunate in having a ready skill that brings them daily into contact with the marvel of the human body, and into conversation with so many different human beings, each one a potential storehouse of experience and knowledge. For Browne, each clinical encounter must have been an opportunity to indulge his curiosity, enthusiasm, and humanitarianism. And just as Browne must have taken inspiration from those he met, he was throughout his writing life a prolific bibliophile, ceaselessly inspired by whatever he was reading. As Coleridge wrote of him: 'A library was a living world to him, and every book a man.'[3] I wonder how much he began to look upon every woman and man as holding the same potential for revelation as a book.

*

Part of being a physician in today's hyperspecialized medical world is that even the most aspirational doctor never going to be an expert in everything. The ocean of possibilities in human suffering is too vast, and the manifestations and origins of illness too plural, for a generalist to be anything other than a dilettante. The ceaseless flow of patients through the clinic, with their infinitude of problems, trains the mind to an acceptance that no matter how long or hard you work you'll never have seen it all. After a few years at the work, this shifts from becoming a frustration of the job to one of its pleasures. A general medical practice provides such immersion in the diversity and multiplicity of humanity that even forty years of practice offers just a few windows onto the numberless ways of living.

The family physician and poet William Carlos Williams recognized that part of its appeal. In his *Old Doc Rivers*, he wrote of one old family physician:

> I'm telling you you never saw an office like it. He had the right idea, he was for humanity—put it any way you like. They'd be sitting all over the place, out in the hall, up the stairs, on the porch, anywhere they could park themselves.[4]

With this depiction of a shabby clinic crowded with the poor, Carlos Williams is alluding to the humility of family practice—something he embraced as a consequence of having stepped off medicine's hierarchy of prestige. And Carlos Williams makes it just as clear that the decision to step off that ladder has its consolations: a feeling of being valued and trusted by people for whom you become a kind of honorary family member.

The relative lowliness of the generalist within the hierarchy of medicine is well known to all GPs and in my experience is variably tolerated or ignored. The anthropologist Cecil Helman worked for many years as a GP, and his book *Suburban Shaman* turns his skills as an anthropologist onto the observation of medical hierarchies in action. He describes attending an educational meeting at a British hospital sometime earlier in his career (the book was published in 2004):

> [The specialists] wear dark suits and shiny black shoes, and several of them are wearing bow-ties. Among them are a few women, in smart charcoal trouser suits and fluffy white blouses, most with tiny earrings and minimal make-up. Every Monday afternoon, they all occupy the first three rows of the big lecture hall in the local hospital, for the weekly Grand Rounds, the academic centre of the week.
>
> Behind the Consultants sit the local general practitioners (one of whom is me)—two rows of tired-looking men and women. We are wearing rougher clothes—tweeds and brogues or other sensible shoes. Unlike the Consultants, our clothing styles are more individual, but the colours are also more muted: country greys and greens and browns, sometimes black or dark blue. Bleepers rest in our pockets or handbags, chirping occasionally like agitated birds. Medical bags rest on our laps or under our seats. All of us family doctors are tired, but alert. Most of us are on-call.[5]

For most modern specialists, just as for the grand physicians of London in Browne's day, general practice is too various in its demands to be considered an elite endeavour. And the work is all the richer for it. To become a specialist is to prefer one organ or disease over all others, with attendant prospects to excel in some unexplored aspect of knowledge. But it doesn't follow that generalists like Browne were therefore unambitious. The physician of a small provincial practice may have other kinds of ambitions, such as those explored in John Berger's landmark study of a country doctor, *A Fortunate Man*: to use medicine as a vehicle to explore the possibilities of humanity.

The kind of modern medical practice that turns no patient or condition away can never be a stranger to humility. Every day it is necessary to exchange coherent letters, and discuss mutual patients, with specialists as diverse as neurosurgeons and nephrologists, podiatrists, and psychodynamic psychotherapists—each of whom have their own language and their own way of understanding the mutual patient's experience. Those encounters I have by phone or letter are a constant reminder of the limitations of my own knowledge, but they also celebrate, in their own way, the breadth of knowledge the profession has obliged me to cultivate over the years. No one has a monopoly on knowledge of the human body or mind, and it often seems to me that GPs are just more honest about that than many specialists. I often act for my patients as an interpreter or guide rather than as the master of my subject.

The parallels between the humility of Christian faith and the humility of caring work in medicine and nursing was well recognized in Browne's Europe: two of his contemporaries in France, Vincent de Paul and Louise de Marillac, were later sainted for their work building hospitals for the sick poor (both died in 1660). The two enjoyed a long, platonic partnership, and in the years subsequent to Browne's own travels through France established nursing as a respectable vocation, with a measure of holiness thrown in. Some of the most advanced French, Swiss, and Italian hospitals today retain a connection to the Church, established at the time when the Church was the only institution to offer care. There's a hint of this attitude in Browne's own approach to his patients, who were at times considered substitutes for Christ, to be served with humble gratitude. Though Browne's humility was tinged with the elitism of his day, his choice of profession, the clinical consultations he offered *gratis* to the indigent of Norwich, even his choice of English rather than Latin for his books, implies a wish to be accessible and open, rather than rarefied and exclusive.

The humility in matters of faith that Browne emphasized, and their connection to his appreciation of the natural world, is evident in the writings of Francis Bacon where it was co-opted to serve his restless search for new ways of understanding. This, from *The History of the Winds,* was published in 1622.

> Therefore, if we have any humility towards the creator; if we have any reverence and esteem of his works; if we have any charity towards men or any desire of relieving their miseries and necessities; if we have any love for natural truths; any aversion to darkness; and any desire of purifying the understanding; mankind are to be most affectionately interested and beseeched to lay aside, at least for a while, their preposterous, *fantastic* and *hypothetical philosophies* (which have *led experience* captive, and childishly triumphed over the works of *God*;) and now at length condescend, and with due submission and veneration, to approach and peruse the *volume of the creation*; dwell some time upon it; and, bringing to the work a mind well purged of opinions, idols and false notions, converse familiarly therein.[6]

Browne was of course more than happy to [con]descend to what Bacon called the *volume of creation,* and his whole approach, on show repeatedly through the *Vulgar Errors,* embodied an attempt to purge his mind of false notions.

The readiness with which he examined the lowliest aspects of nature with a clear vision can be seen in his admiration of insects. In *Urn Burial* he writes of his fascination with the funereal habits of ants ('pismires') and bees:

> They that are so thick skinned as still to credit the story of the phoenix, may say something for animal burning: More serious conjectures find some examples of sepulture in elephants, cranes, the sepulchral cells of pismires and the practice of bees; which civil society carries out their dead, and have exequies, if not interments.[7]

And in *Religio Medici*, Browne enthuses about how much more there is to marvel at in the lives of the spiders and insects, observable in his Norfolk garden, than there is in the megafauna of Africa or Asia:

> Indeed what reason may not go to school to the wisdom of bees, ants, and spiders? Ruder heads stand amazed at those prodigious pieces of nature, whales, elephants, dromedaries, and camels; these I confess, are the colossus and majestic pieces of her hand; but in these narrow engines there is more curious mathematics, and the civility of these little citizens more neatly sets forth the wisdom of their maker.[8]

*

Accepting Browne's humility in matters of faith, and in matters of knowledge, his choice of a provincial medical practice hints at a third way that he understood the importance of the virtue: humility in social relations. He clearly believed in an elitism of the mind, and though he pronounced himself humble, you can hardly imagine him cleaning out the toilets. Claire Preston wrote in *Thomas Browne and the Writings of Early Modern Science* that *Vulgar Errors* was of all his books the one most obviously written in a 'low style' intended to appeal to a wide audience. Preston explicitly draws out how much Browne owed to Francis Bacon in this respect: 'The choice of the vernacular, moreover, is a thoroughly Baconian one: to revile secrecy in learning by expressing it in common languages was to oppose the subtle obscurities of Scholasticism and the extravagant occultism of alchemy; it was to promote the utility of learning for the common good.'[9] Although Browne cultivated an elitism that was intellectual, and engaged in social relations across the spectrum of society, he believed that the performance of humility was essential not only to be true to his faith, but to advance through the caste hierarchies of seventeenth-century England. In *A Letter to a Friend* he was candid about the extent to which this must involve deception:

> Be substantially great in yourself and more than you appear unto others; and let the world be deceived in you as they are in the lights of heaven. Hang early plummets upon the heels of pride, and let ambition have but an epicycle or narrow circuit in you.[10]

Ambition was laudable, but must be controlled, and one must be discreet about manifesting it. True happiness is to be found in a circle of trusted friends, and hell is right here on earth, in the torments of a bad conscience:

> Bless me in this life with but peace of my conscience, command of my affections, the love of Thyself and my dearest friends, and I shall be happy enough to pity Cæsar. These are, O Lord, the humble desires of my most reasonable ambition, and all I dare call happiness on earth.[11]

His son Edward seems to have owed his success among the upper reaches of London society in part to the fame of Browne senior, as well as to liberal amounts of fatherly advice—Edward was Fellow of the Royal Society in his thirties, President of the

Royal College of Physicians in his sixties, and was honoured by being made a physician to the Royal Court. Among Browne's many paternal recommendations was that Edward's performance of humility should always be allied with restless industry: 'Be careful of yourself and temperate, that you may be able to go through your practice; for to attain to the getting of a thousand pounds a year requires no small labour of body and mind.'[12]

*

One of Browne's strangest books is an exploration of figures of five in nature, a pattern he sees everywhere and which her refers to as 'the quincunx'. In Samuel Johnson's *Life of Browne,* I was delighted to find the following passage:

> it is a perpetual triumph of fancy to expand a scanty theme, to raise glittering ideas from obscure properties, and to produce to the world an object of wonder to which nature had contributed little. To this ambition, perhaps, we owe the Frogs of HOMER, the Gnat and the Bees of VIRGIL, the Butterfly of SPENSER, the Shadow of WOWERUS, and the Quincunx of BROWNE.[13]

For Johnson, the virtue of Browne's writings is expressed by his care and wonder over the most modest observations of the natural world, from patterns seen in botany to the industry of the bee. The conviction that arrogance is a vice is one that infuses all of Browne's work, and he took to heart that humility insisted upon by Bacon—the humility he suggests we all should all feel before the magnificence of Creation. At the same time, he clearly recognized the importance of performing self-effacement if one was to advance socially at the bear pit of the Restoration court. But of all the expressions of humility that I have gleaned from my reading of his works it's his satisfaction in work with the poor and his choice of a provincial general practice that I recognize most keenly, as well as the emphasis he placed on the more humble aspects of medical practice which remains, even in our technomedical twenty-first century, the hit-and-miss art of relieving human suffering wherever and in whomever it occurs.

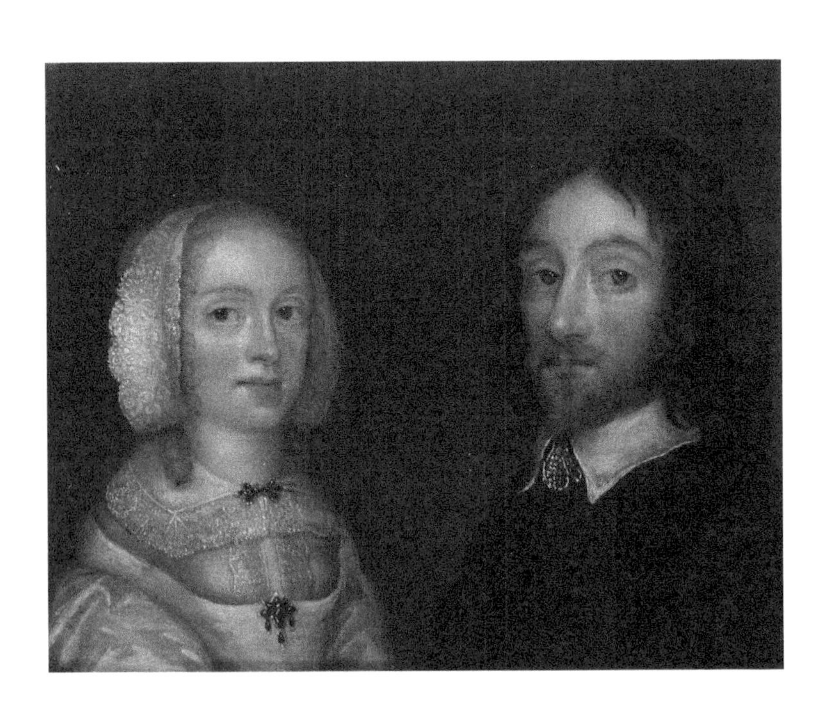

6

MISOGYNY

Unto the woman he said, I will greatly multiply thy sorrow and thy conception; in sorrow thou shalt bring forth children; and thy desire shall be to thy husband, and he shall rule over thee.

Genesis 3: 16

The whole world was made for man, but the twelfth part of man for woman: Man is the whole world, and the breath of God; woman the rib and crooked piece of man.

Religio Medici 2:9

The literary record is half-silenced; in seventeenth-century Europe far fewer women than men were literate, and far fewer ever reached positions of intellectual respect never mind influence. Browne's wife Dorothy Mileham was, however, highly literate, loved, and respected for her intellectual and organizational abilities as much as for her domestic ones.

Queen Elizabeth spoke to the pervasive misogyny of England when she said, 'I know I have the body of a weak and feeble woman but I have the heart and stomach of a king.'* Female dramatists had some success: in England, notably Aphra Behn, who was born when Browne was in his mid-thirties, and in the Spain of the 1630s, Maria de Zayas y Sotomayor. Her Spain was one bloated with Bolivian silver and Mexican gold, and she wrote with fury of how women in that society of almost unimaginable wealth were

* In her speech to the troops at Tilbury.

yet kept ignorant, denied education. One of her novels gives voice to the frustration that she and her peers endured:

> Why vain legislators of the world, do you tie our hands so that we cannot take vengeance? Because of your mistaken ideas about us, you render us powerless and deny us access to pen and sword. Isn't our soul the same as a man's soul?[1]

Padua wouldn't have its first woman graduate until years after Browne was there, and so his formative years, intellectually speaking, were in an entirely male environment. It was only in the latter part of the century, with the growth of literary salons in Paris, then London, that there began to be the opportunity for men and women to meet as equals in an atmosphere of intellectual encouragement. Beyond London, Katherine Philips's *Society of Friendship*, established in Cardigan, Wales, in the late 1640s and transplanted to Dublin in 1662 (the year Browne was asked to intervene in a witchcraft trial), was a place for women and men to share discussions of poetry and ideas freely. In 1664, Philips went to London, where she died of smallpox (the subject of Browne's Leiden thesis) and that same year her poems were published 'surreptitiously' as *Poems, By the Incomparable Mrs K. P.*

That was the year Browne's son Thomas was beginning his service in the British Navy, and Edward left for his own tour of the Continent: Paris, Genoa, Bologna, Padua, and Venice. Browne's daughter Anne was married, and had become a mother. Browne's other daughters appear as brief mentions in the family correspondence between the men, and only occasionally as senders or recipients of letters in their own right. Betty, the daughter who would read to Browne in his old age, is described by Edward as particularly gifted. One wonders what she might have made of her talent in a world where women and men were equally encouraged to pursue their abilities and enthusiasms not only as a pastime, but as a means to making a living. 'Though I make many journeys, yet I am confident that your pen and pencil are greater travellers', Edward wrote to her; 'How many fine plains do they pass over, and how many hills, woods, seas do they design? You have a fine way of not only seeing but making a world; and whilst you set still, how many miles doth your hand travel!'[2]

*

Browne claimed in *Religio Medici* that 'I borrow not the rules of my Religion from *Rome* or *Geneva*, but the dictates of my own reason.' But he clearly thinks of women as less capable than men—a position entirely cultural in its origins, with little in it of the application of reason. He wonders why God is said to have created woman as a helper for man, because in terms of muscular strength, 'it had been fitter to have made another man.' He assumed the only help offered was 'unto generation' because, though Adam must by his reasoning have included all human nature and thus both sexes, 'Hermaphrodites, although they include the parts of both sexes, and may be sufficiently potent in either; yet unto a conception require a separated sex, and cannot impregnate themselves.'[3]

There are many further examples of his muddled thinking on sexual difference: 'The whole world was made for man, but the twelfth part of man for woman.'[4] These early beliefs coexisted in a mind that as we've discussed, was entirely at ease with paradox, and which was convinced that, physiologically speaking, there is little difference between women and men. He considers carefully the several reliable stories he has heard of women changing into men, and though he's aware of stories of the reverse occurring in some animals, he doesn't know of any male-to-female transition of sex in human beings:

> As for the mutation of sexes or transition into one another, we cannot deny it in hares, it being observable in man. For hereof, beside Empedocles or Tiresias, there are not a few examples; and though very few, or rather none which have emasculated or turned women, yet very many who from an esteem or reality of being women have infallibly proved men; some at the first point of the menstrous eruptions, some in the day of their marriage, others many years after.[5,†]

Browne's was an era in which the Bible was widely interpreted as literal truth (as it still is in some quarters today), but he's aware of scripture's many contradictions, in particular that part of Genesis which claims first that Eve was created from the rib of Adam, and then that man and woman were created simultaneously by God, then separated—an inconsistency that in Jewish lore gives rise to the myth of Lilith. Quoting Montaigne, Browne points out that not all human communities complain of pain in childbirth. He notices that Adam volunteered to eat the forbidden fruit, while Eve had to be tricked by the serpent into taking it—raising the question of whether she might in fact have been more far-sighted and virtuous than he. Browne is altogether perplexed by the Fall and expulsion from Eden, and you've the sense, on reading him, that he doesn't quite believe it: Adam's gullibility was 'very strange and inexcusable ... especially, if as some affirm, he was the wisest of all men since; or if, as others have conceived, he was

† Browne is almost certainly talking of intersex conditions here such as Congenital Adrenal Hyperplasia and Testicular Feminisation, now known and understood as hormonal conditions and grouped together as 'disorders of sexual differentiation.'

not ignorant of the fall of the angels, and had thereby example and punishment to deter him'.[6] Eve shouldn't be blamed; she was 'inveigled' with 'allurements', and as a consequence her 'posterity has been deluded ever since'.

Any student of anatomy who has paid the slightest bit of attention knows that men and women have an equal number of ribs, twenty-four, or twelve on each side. And the last couple of decades have seen a flurry of scholarly articles suggesting that the Hebrew word *tzela* doesn't mean rib anyway, but any kind of supportive bone, and that what the Genesis story is doing in mythical terms is supplying an explanation of why human beings alone among great apes lack a penis bone, or baculum.[7] From this perspective Eve wasn't made from a rib at all; the story is implying that the creation of men and women was made possible through human development away from the anatomical peculiarities of apes. Browne thought a fair amount about ribs, not least about which of Adam or Eve would be resurrected with their shared rib at the Apocalypse. Here he is describing an anatomical demonstration by the great anatomist Realdo Colombo at the University of Pisa (Colombo was incidentally the first anatomist to notice the clitoris, and was denounced by Vesalius for granting it greater importance than the latter felt it deserved):

> That a man hath one rib less then a woman, is a common conceit derived from the History of Genesis, wherein it stands delivered, that Eve was framed out of a rib of Adam; whence 'tis concluded the sex of man still wants that rib our Father lost in Eve. And this is not only passant with the many, but was urged against Columbus in an Anatomy of his at Pisa, where having prepared the skeleton of a woman that chanced to have thirteen ribs on one side, there

> arose a party that cried him down, and even unto oaths affirmed, this was the rib wherein a woman exceeded. Were this true, it would ocularly silence that dispute out of which side Eve was framed.[8]

*

Browne's statement as a young bachelor, in *Religio Medici,* that 'we might procreate, like trees, without conjunction, or that there were any way to perpetuate the World without this trivial and vulgar way of coition'[9] has occasioned much sniggering over the years among Browne's readers. Not least among those sniggerers was Samuel Johnson, who wrote that news of Browne's marriage to Dorothy Mileham couldn't help but draw the 'raillery of contemporary wits',[10] and who made fun of the famous writer for his evident change of heart. At thirty he'd written of sexual intercourse that it 'is the foolishest act a wise man commits in all his life'; six years later he was married, and within at most two more (the specific dates of either Browne's marriage or the births of his children are unrecorded), he was a father. Samuel Taylor Coleridge, always indulgent and enthusiastic in his notes on reading Browne, was puzzled by this odd antipathy to sex: 'He says, he is a Batchelor, but he talks as if he had been a married man, & married to a Woman who did not love him, & whom he did not love. Taken by itself, no doubt, the act is foolish, & debasing. But what a misery is contained in those words, "taken by itself?"'[11]

On reading *The Rings of Saturn,* a book animated and threaded through with reflections, quotations, and revelations from Browne's works, I've wondered whether Sebald's disgusted account of coming upon a couple making love on a beach near Covehithe in Suffolk is specifically intended to echo that 'foolish & debasing' perspective on sex offered by the younger Browne.

> A couple lay down there, in the bottom of the pit, as I thought: a man stretched full length over another body of which nothing was visible but the legs, spread and angled. In the startled moment when that image went through me, which lasted an eternity, it seemed as if the man's feet twitched like those of one just hanged. Now, though, he lay still, and the woman too was still and motionless. Misshapen, like some great mollusc washed ashore, they lay there, to all appearances a single being, a many limbed, two-headed monster that had drifted in from far out at sea, the last of a prodigious species, its life ebbing from it with each breath expired through its nostrils. Filled with consternation, I stood up once more, shaking as if it were that first time in my life that I had got to my feet, and left the place, which seemed fearsome to me now, taking the path that descended from the cliff-top to where the beach spread out on the southerly side.[12]

'Misshapen' 'many limbed' 'motionless' 'monster', which 'twitches' like 'one just hanged'; this is an abomination, not an act of love, or of the generation that so fascinated Browne, who would have preferred that humans procreate by means of stamens and pollen. In the same vein that Browne wonders whether, for a 'help' in the garden of Eden, God might not have more effectively furnished Adam with another man, he seems to be resigned to the existence of women, at least until his own marriage occurred. Following that marriage, his writings express a physician's detachment about the mechanics of sex, of penises and testicles, vaginas and wombs, yet marvel at the mysteries of fertility without ever again expressing distaste.

*

'I am, I confess, naturally inclined to that which misguided zeal terms superstition',[13] he wrote, and it's that superstition which provides one of the most chilling examples of the misogyny of seventeenth-century England—the torture, trial, and murder of women accused of witchcraft. For the Browne of *Religio Medici*, it is beyond question that there exists a hierarchy of creatures ascending from matter to plants to animals to humans to spirits, or angels, and it's in the realm of spirits that he claims that witchcraft does its evil work. He knew the Old Testament well, and was aware that in the book of Samuel, King Saul is described as consulting with the witch of Endor to discern the future.[14] For Browne, biblical stories of witchcraft meant taking their existence for granted, because he prioritized scriptural over empirical proof. 'I have ever believed, and do now know, that there are witches: they that doubt of these, do not only deny them, but spirits; and are obliquely and upon consequence a sort not of infidels, but atheists.'[15] It's an odd position to hold for one who remains so carefully balanced in all of his other opinions regarding matters of faith—to question the existence of witches would be for him to question the existence of God. 'Of all the delusions wherewith he deceives mortality, there is not any that puzzles me more than the Legerdemain [trickery] of Changelings',[16] he goes on, 'I do not credit those transformations of reasonable creatures into beasts, or that the Devil hath a power to transpeciate a man into a Horse.' After all, it's written that the devil tempted Jesus to use his spiritual powers to convert stones into bread.

In a series of articles for *The Guardian* in 2003, Roz Kaveney puzzled over Browne's bizarre adherence to witchcraft as an empirical truth. Kaveney wrote:

> He did one very bad thing that we know about, one which seems peculiarly inconsistent with his elevation of empirical reason as a partner to faith. He appeared as an expert witness in a witchcraft

> trial in Bury St Edmunds, and testified that some young girls who, he said, undoubtedly had things medically wrong with them, were also bewitched. He also mentioned reports of a similar case in Denmark. It's been claimed that his testimony swayed the jurors into sending two old women to the gallows, though a town that had been caught up a few years earlier in the murderous frenzy of Matthew Hopkins, witchfinder-general, hardly needed much persuading. In the end, Browne was complicit in judicial murder because he regarded witchcraft as a real thing, because it was in scripture and in the news reports—when we praise his sweet reasonableness, we need to remember its limits.[17]

Like Kaveney and many others, I've been dismayed and disappointed by this episode in Browne's biography. But it's also true to say that Browne himself never wrote about the trial, and we only know of his involvement because of a description published twenty years after the fact, in 1682 ('A Tryal of Witches at the Assizes Held at Bury St. Edmonds').

The trial was of two women, Rose Cullender and Amy Denny, who stood accused of bewitching Elizabeth Pacy (11) and Deborah Pacy (9), the two daughters of a prominent businessman from Lowestoft. But in addition to that allegation, fourteen other counts against the women emerged arising from accusations made by several different families. Some of the events were said to have taken place several years prior, in the 1650s: Denny was accused of sickening a boy called William by breastfeeding him, and to have brought about the death of a girl called Elizabeth. Browne wasn't involved in the case, hadn't seen any of the victims as patients, and seems to have been asked to give a general

'Opinion' at short notice. The report, two-decades later, said of Browne that he related an anecdote:

> That in Denmark there had been lately a great discovery of witches, who used the very same way of afflicting persons, by conveying pins into them, and crooked as these pins were, with needles and nails. And his opinion was that the devil in such cases did work upon the bodies of men and women, upon a natural foundation, (that is) to stir up, and excite such humours super-abounding in their bodies to a great excess, whereby he did in an extraordinary manner afflict them with such distempers as their bodies were most subject to, as particularly appeared in these children; for he conceived, that these swooning fits were natural, and nothing else but what they call the Mother, but only heightened to a great excess by the subtilty of the devil, co-operating with the malice of these which we term witches, at whose instance he does these villainies.[18]

And so what emerges is that Browne didn't condemn these women at all, in fact he said that the children were simply victims of 'the Mother' i.e. hysteria. 'Hysteria' is of course an atavistic, misogynistic term, but the illness that it describes is entirely real, and most modern doctors, myself included, have seen plenty examples of it. If we believe the report, the girls seem to have suffered what would now be called a *sociogenic* or *functional neurological* illness—an entirely natural reaction to a complex state of mind exacerbated by the delirious atmosphere of the trial (Elizabeth Pacy was shown to swoon, when blindfolded, when touched by a neutral person, just as if she had been touched by a witch). But with Browne's testimony—that these natural swooning fits could quite possibly have been 'heightened' by the devil acting maliciously—an opportunity to save these women's lives was missed. Both were hung on the gallows shortly afterwards, on 17 March.

In his biography of Browne, Reid Barbour doesn't excuse Browne's lack of zeal in expounding just how much doubt must always surround such cases, but thoughtfully lists some of the ways in which Browne would have had to be very careful about making such an intervention.[19] First, the kind of medicine he practised was largely believed to overlap with magic, and the common people often suspected physicians of something akin to witchcraft. Second, there was a suspicion that the devil was behind any attempts to prove the non-existence of witches, in order to do further mischief. Third, witch trials were almost always instigated by powerful, moneyed citizens against poor, isolated, and elderly women, and each trial constituted the culmination of months or even years of opaque local tensions that a visiting physician such as Browne would have had little knowledge of. Fourth, there was hardly any consensus on the point at which possession, which was presumed to require exorcism, shaded into witchcraft, which required solely the elucidation and punishment of the culpable witch.

Hippocrates had said that epileptic seizures were simply a disorder of the brain, not the 'sacred disease' of spiritual possession, but that Greek perspective was complicated by the several New Testament episodes in which seizures are considered to be straightforward examples of possession. The final problem for a physician like Browne, says Barbour, was that Francis Bacon had at the close of the sixteenth century insisted that 'new philosophers' should examine carefully cases like witchcraft, where natural events seemed to shade into the otherworldly, or 'preternatural'.

What then are we to make of Browne's misogyny? He was a man of his times, who knew better than most how few differences there really are between masculine and feminine physiology.

Browne devotes substantial space in *Vulgar Errors* to debunking the traditional belief that women, when drowned, float prone, while men float supine. He shows how the idea that this might in some way have arisen to protect female modesty is absurd, and wonders whether the tradition arose because of male and female variations in typical distribution of fat:

> If so, then Men with great bellies will float downward, and only Callipygæ ['beautiful buttocks'] and Women largely composed behind, upward. But anatomists observe, that to make the larger cavity for the Infant, the haunch bones in Women, and consequently the parts appendant are more protuberant then they are in Men. They who ascribe the cause unto the breasts of Women, take not away the doubt; for they resolve not why children float downward, who are included in that sex, though not in the reason alleged.[20]

Actually, none of Browne's reasoning is correct—all humans float largely head down when drowned, depending on the air content of their bodies, because of the weight and density of the skull.

Browne believed transitions between genders were possible, and that the biblical excuses for men having been granted power to rule over women were thin to non-existent. The provincial world he moved in saw women constrained and limited at every juncture of their lives, and though in northern Italy he would have encountered or heard of female physicians, their very exceptionalism seems to have reinforced prejudice against the education of women, rather than weakened it. He stewed in a morass of misconceived ideas about the devil's malevolent influence on humanity, and on women in particular, because of another perennial misconception: that women were uniquely vulnerable to 'hysteria'. Far more likely is that that the social circumstances of women pushed them into manifesting its symptoms more frequently than men.

*

One of the last written accounts of spending time with Thomas Browne occurs in a letter from Lord Yarmouth, written to his wife after visiting Browne at his home on the market square in Norwich. The letter describes who else was in the house when he called by.[21] According to Reid Barbour, Yarmouth painted a picture of Browne contented, and surrounded by the many women in his life. There was a Mrs Peirce, her daughter, Mrs Needham, the wife of Colonel Harbord, and presumably Browne's wife Dorothy. Barbour concludes:

> This image of Browne resonates with the prospect that in a world driven (for Edward) by ambition, for the late Thomas Jr. by military valor, and increasingly for masculine political culture by bitter rivalry and partisanship, it was the women in his life who surrounded the aging physician with the civility, flexibility, and good-heartedness for which he had always longed.

Stories that have emerged from Browne's marriage constitute one of the strongest arguments in his favour—that for all the misogyny in his writing, he and Dorothy were able to sustain as equal a partnership as was possible given the times in which they lived. Dorothy was characterized by one of Browne's earliest biographers, John Whitefoot, as 'a Lady of such a Symmetrical Proportion to her Worthy Husband, both in the Graces of her Body and Mind, that they seemed to come together by a kind of

Natural Magnetism'. When Browne died, he left everything to Dorothy, and granted her executive power over all his estate (the will was prepared three years before his death).

The author of Dorothy's epitaph is unknown, but she died three years after her husband. It's there in St Peter Mancroft in Norwich still, engraved on a memorial stone of the north wall of the church. And although the epitaph alludes to her qualities as a wife and mother, its focus on her intellect is unusual for the period. It may have been written by her son Edward, but if not, was certainly approved of by her four surviving children:

Reader! thou maist beleive this sacred Stone;
It is not common Dust, thou tread'st upon;
'Tis hallowed Earth, all that is left below,
Of what the World admir'd, and honor'd too,
The Prison of a bright celestial Mind,
Too spacious to be longer here confin'd;
Which after all that Vertue could inspire,
Or unaffected Piety require;
In all the noblest Offices of Life,
Of tenderest Benefactress, Mother, Wife,
To those serene Abodes above, is flown,
To be adorn'd with an immortal Crown.

A

Brief Account

OF SOME

TRAVELS

IN

HUNGARIA,	*AUSTRIA,*
SERVIA,	*STYRIA,*
BULGARIA,	*CARINTHIA,*
MACEDONIA,	*CARNIOLA,*
THESSALY,	and *FRIULI.*

As alſo

Some Obſervations on the *Gold*, *Silver*, *Copper*, *Quick-ſilver Mines*, *Baths*, and *Mineral Waters* in thoſe parts:

With the

Figures of ſome Habits and Remarkable places.

By *EDWARD BROWN* M. D.
of the College of *LONDON*, Fellow of the *R. Society*,
and Phyſician in Ordinary to His MAJESTY.

LONDON,
Printed by *T. R.* for *Benj. Tooke*, and are to be Sold at the
Sign of the *Ship* in St. *Pauls* Church-yard, 1673.

7

MOBILITY

To a man of active mind too long attachment to one college is apt to breed self-satisfaction, to narrow his outlook, to foster a local spirit, and to breed senility.

William Osler *The Fixed Period*

...to attempt perpetual motions, and engines whose revolutions might out-last the exemplary mobility, and out-measure time itself.

Vulgar Errors 5:19

The English writer Bruce Chatwin described religion as a travel guide for settlers, as if those who travel widely have too much experience of plurality of belief and human habits to set much store by the kinds of received truths that buttress so much of what passes for religion. The word arises, after all, from the Latin *religare*, 'to bind', and it might be expected that those people who are most mobile, unbound by the obligation to stay home, would be the most lax in matters of faith.

For the first thirty years or so of life Browne travelled more than was common for his time. He wrote of his 'simpling in Cheapside' as a child—to simple was to gather medicinal plants—whether through the fields and meadows then still extant around the part of London where he lived, or among the stalls selling herbs in the markets isn't clear. After the death of his father he came very close to suffering an unwelcome downward social mobility, but a court case secured his inheritance from his mother and her new husband, and facilitated his education in Winchester, then Oxford. As a young man of seventeen he made a journey around Ireland with his landowning, militarist stepfather, was shipwrecked, kidnapped, and had to be ransomed (for sixpence) by the parishioners of his London church of St Michael de Querne. He later wrote some mediocre poetry about the storm in which his ship was overwhelmed, mentioning it both in letters to his children, and in *Religio Medici*: 'I have been shipwrackt, yet am not enemy with the Sea or Winds.'[1] It's disappointing to have no record of what Browne thought of the colonialist project of the English in Ireland of that time. For such a privileged boy, a horseback journey around Ireland must have offered startling revelations of different ways of living, although Samuel Johnson oddly dismissed the trip: 'Ireland had, at that time, very little to offer to the observation of a man of letters.'[2]

Following his graduation from Oxford, Browne set out on what would become the longest journey he ever undertook: the grand tour that took in studies at Montpellier, Padua, and Leiden, between 1631 and 1634. On returning to England he went north to Yorkshire, to take up a role as a kind of apprentice to a country physician. The transition from an elite university to a backward country practice must have been stark, and it's there that he seems to have written the first draft of *Religio Medici* for circulation among his friends. If Chatwin is correct about religion being a travel guide for settlers, then that book's restless sparring with faith could be seen as Browne's reconciliation with the idea of settling down to a more binding kind of a life.

From Halifax he moved to Norwich, where he stayed until the end of his life (from the age of thirty-two until his death at seventy-seven), but Browne never did 'settle down', in terms of the restiveness of his imagination. In his correspondence, in his choice of reading, in the horseback home visits he made around Norfolk, he never cloistered himself. He was the first editor of his son Edward's travel journals (Edward Browne pleased his father when he disclosed just how often, on his travels in Southern and Eastern Europe, he was fêted for being the son of the author of *Religio Medici*). In later life, his favourite daughter Betty would read to him, and a list of their preferred books survives: Rycaut on the history of the Ottoman emperors, travel accounts of China, Turkey, Naples, Venice, *Plutarch's Lives, Foxe's Book of Martyrs,* among many others. He read the 'Journall of captaine Abel Jansen Tasman' about his voyage to the recently discovered continent that would later be called Australia, and carried on a long correspondence about Iceland with a Lutheran minister there, gleaning information that he submitted in 1663 to the Royal Society as 'An Account of Island, alias Ice-land'. The Society had been founded only a couple of years before, and one of its original twelve members, the great chemist Robert Boyle, wrote a book about ice that drew on just such anecdotal accounts (though he complained that, to get information about icebergs, glaciers, and the differing modes of freezing of salt and fresh water, it was necessary to labour through 'melancholy accounts of storms and distresses, and ice, and bears, and foxes'[3]). From his study in Norwich, Browne travelled far in his imagination, and in his memory, and as long as he practised medicine he never ceased from travelling through the landscapes of his patients' lives. His great admirer Henry David Thoreau might be said to have adopted a similar perspective when he wrote:

> I, on my side, require of every writer, first or last, a simple and sincere account of his own life, and not merely what he has heard of

other men's lives; some such account as he would send to his kindred from a distant land; for if he has lived sincerely, it must have been in a distant land to me.*[4]

*

Lytton Strachey imagined Browne's writings as redolent of a kind of mystical exoticism, as if only in an oriental (and orientalist) context would his talents best be revealed:

> It is interesting—or at least amusing—to consider what are the most appropriate places in which different authors should be read. Pope is doubtless at his best in the midst of a formal garden, Herrick in an orchard, and Shelley in a boat at sea, Sir Thomas Browne demands, perhaps, a more exotic atmosphere. One could read him floating down the Euphrates, or past the shores of Arabia; and it would be pleasant to open *Vulgar Errors* in Constantinople, or to get by heart a chapter of the *Christian Morals* between the paws of a Sphinx. In England, the most fitting background for his strange ornament must surely be some habitation consecrated to learning, some university which still smells of antiquity, and has learned the habit of repose.[5]

That Browne's prose is transporting, exotic, evocative of voyages and strange expeditions, was something E.M. Forster too celebrated in his story *The Celestial Omnibus*, in which a young boy follows a signpost up an alley that purports to lead 'To Heaven', and is confronted by a carriage with two horses, the driver of which is Browne. The boy has no money to pay for his ticket, so offers Browne his watch as a substitute, but is refused. Though an

* Though Thoreau's contemporary in Massachusetts Emily Dickinson read Browne, there's no explicit record of what she thought of his books, though many have thought her own work influenced by them. On 25 April 1862 she wrote to Colonel Thomas Wentworth Higginson: 'For poets, I have Keats, and Mr. and Mrs Browning. For prose, Mr. Ruskin, Sir Thomas Browne, and the Revelations.'

admirer of Browne, Forster has some fun at his expense, parroting the dense allusiveness of his prose: 'Tickets on this line', replies Browne, 'whether single or return, can be purchased by coinage from no terrene mint. And a chronometer, though it had solaced the vigils of Charlemagne, or measured the slumbers of Laura, can acquire by no mutation the double-cake that charms the fangless Cerberus of Heaven!'[6] Forster's addition of an exclamation mark is the only wrong note in the dialogue. Browne invites the boy up onto the box to ride alongside him, and the horses canter out over a flaming rainbow that licks at their wheels but allows them to ascend over a gulf of clouds into a new land of the imagination, where Achilles and the Duchess of Malfi are real, and where the air is filled with the melody of Wagner's *Rhinegold*. Browne's isn't the only omnibus travelling to this land: Forster describes other carriages driven by Shelley, and a scowling, inscrutable Dante.

'As a healer of bodies, I had scant success', Browne says to Forster's boy when he is asked about his profession 'But as a healer of the spirit I have succeeded beyond my hopes and my deserts. For though my draughts were not better nor subtler than those of other men, yet, by reason, of the cunning goblets wherein I offered them, the queasy soul was ofttimes tempted to sip and be refreshed.'

This is literature as vessel, as vehicle, as vicarious experience, as balm and even as convalescence, just as 'a change is as good as a rest', and for the same reason the Victorian sanatoria were built on the highest slopes among the purest air.

*

In the 1990s, Edinburgh medical school promoted two kinds of travelling for the benefit of its students. For those taking a year from strictly medical studies to study for an Honours BSc, there was the possibility of an exchange programme with Leiden University. Then for the final-year students, there were four months of 'elective' in which it was obligatory to seek placements elsewhere. We were encouraged to be creative, to build connections with hospitals and universities anywhere in the world. Fiji, Barbados, Chicago, Sydney, Paris, Montreal, Beirut, and Johannesburg are some of the places I remember as destinations of my peers. There were grants to which we could apply to pay for the air fares, and most of the placements themselves were offered entirely free of charge, as contributions towards the sharing of knowledge, and perhaps as offerings to the gift economy of a worldwide family of physicians. Many who hosted such students had links to Edinburgh, or had themselves qualified there.

At that time there was little in the way of internet contact with the hospitals; more traditional methods of communication were required. In the administration office at the entranceway of the old Victorian medical school building there was a fat red folder filled with testimonials and addresses from Addis Ababa to Zaragoza. Students were encouraged to find a quiet time to look through the folder, jot down the addresses of hospitals that appealed, and write to them.

The first part of my elective was in East Africa, where I learned something of white privilege, the many legacies of colonialism, and to never take the kind of hospitals, pharmacies, and clinics I'd been trained in for granted. But I also learned how transformative the most simple of medical interventions could be, how cheaply they could be effected, and how the world and the ways of human beings were vaster and more limitlessly various than I had ever before conceived them. I became accustomed to the practice of medicine as it was once in my own country, the stench and filth of it: babies dying of tetanus, of malaria, able to live only a year or two at most. There were many firsts for me: a child with her face swollen to double its size with lymphoma, many toddlers whose bellies were blown up with fluid caused by a diet of pure starch. I remember a girl of about thirteen, with burns across her face, arms, and neck from falling into a fire. Her cheap dressings were soaked with pus, and she was unable to afford the honey dressings that the nurses recommended. Across the bandages of her neck, face, and within her wounds teemed thousands of tiny ants, intent on retrieving organic material from the slough of her wounds. She was stone-faced, silent at the doctor's questions. No relatives came to visit.

To my shame I don't remember offering to pay for those honey dressings myself. Perhaps I was stifled by what I interpreted as the impatience and brusque hostility of the doctor who led the rounds. As a foreign student, new to the continent, I felt I had little to offer, and that it would have been arrogant or in some other way inappropriate to intervene. But I began to learn, I hope, from the relative privilege of my experience, without becoming a voyeur.

That placement was a lesson in the misery inherent in so many lives, the vital part that can be played by good and affordable medicine, the importance of compassion but also the danger of it, when fellow feeling becomes so strong that it begins to paralyse and overwhelm.

*

Browne's liberation in having wandered through Europe for his education is something valorized again and again in the literature of his century, not just in order to be schooled in the finest minds of European medical thought, but to broaden one's outlook and be exposed to many different customs, languages, attitudes. 'Those national repugnances do not touch me, nor do I behold with prejudice the French, Italian, Spaniard, and Dutch', Browne wrote in *Religio Medici*, 'but where I find their actions in balance with my countrymen's, I honour, love, and embrace them in the same degree. I was born in the eighth climate, but seem to be framed and constellated unto all. I am no plant that will not prosper out of a garden: all places, all airs make unto me one country.'[7]

Browne had read Paracelsus very closely—a physician who revolutionized medicine more than a century before Browne's lifetime, and who as an alchemist but also as a doctor joined the Venetian army and travelled in Egypt, Russia, and Arabia. Paracelsus's enquiries and observations ultimately led him to reject the theory of medicine that had stood largely unchallenged for almost two thousand years, that of health being dependent on the balance between four humours, and wrote, 'I have not been ashamed to learn from tramps, butchers and barbers.' With such an open mind, he took knowledge wherever he could, more from marketplaces than from dusty libraries. The same could be said of Browne, who implied that it was travel that had inculcated in him his notorious toleration—a rare quality in the England of the Civil War years. 'I wonder not at the French for their dishes of frogs, snails, and toadstools; nor at the Jews for locusts and grasshoppers; but being amongst them, make them my common viands; and I find them agree with my stomach as well as theirs. I could digest a salad gathered in a churchyard as well as in a garden.'[8]

Twenty years after Browne left Leiden, the physician William Hammond wrote, 'The profession I have now undertaken, gathers like a snowball in rolling; and tis apparent that our greatest doctors in Physic, have been those, who by the advantage of travelling, have viewed, compared and digested the several practices of most of the European physicians.' Though he journeyed around Europe more than a century after Paracelsus, Browne was a forerunner of many later physicians who did the same and who are now more celebrated for their mastery of the profession than he ever was. He studied in Padua, but there's no memorial to his time there; the university does, however, still commemorate those Northern European physicians who ultimately contributed more to the advancement of medicine: William Harvey for example, who was the first to publish a theory of the circulation of the blood, and the Dane Thomas Bartholin, who said of travel:

> In our age such great usefulness redounds to the physician from his travels that no one puts much faith in the authority of a physician who has not set foot outside his native land, and although each may have at home in abundance those things which are necessary for medical instruction, nevertheless they ought to be strengthened or increased by a comparison with things abroad.[9]

Bartholin promoted travel for the aspiring physician, but he also adored it for its own sake. 'There is a vast delight and pleasure in gazing upon foreign lands and fields, mountains and rivers, observing the benignity of nature's variety everywhere.' Though the journey was to be enjoyed for its own sake, the wise physician should be forever observant of different customs and traditions of healing, alert to gauging whether any could be adapted for use at home. He asked young physicians to observe 'the different conditions of the sick in homes and in hospitals with their great number of beds, which can readily be seen here and there, examining the methods for treating the patients, enjoying the conversation of the learned men and calling forth their experiences, and visiting the laboratories, the furnaces of the chemists, the pharmacies and unguent shops'. Bartholin quotes extensively from Galen, who recommended not only that the sick should travel (in *De Icteri Cura* he recommended horseback riding for those suffering bodily weakness) but that trainee physicians should journey extensively to see for themselves the many ways there are of practising their art.

*

The second part of my own student elective was cancelled at short notice, and so from the one available computer terminal at the East African hospital I sent what was still called an 'electronic mail' to a friend, Vivek Muthurangu, now a professor of cardiac physiology, but then a student on a general medical placement in New York.

New York felt like an intoxication, but I'd left it too late to set up any clinical placements. Vivek and I slept in the dormitory of a hostel on East 27th street, our bunkroom shared with a succession of pilgrims and hopefuls from Kentucky and Kansas, Ireland and Israel, none of whom were interested in the sights of the city, but in waking early, putting on their best suits, and stepping out with bundles of CVs to find work.

When it was clear that no hospital would accept me, I took a train to Bethesda and presented myself at the National Institute of Mental Health. I'd secured an invitation from Mortimer Mishkin, one of the world's authorities on the way the brain makes and retrieves memories, and with the generosity of one who believes in a global fraternity of the mind, he had invited me to come and meet him. On arrival at Mishkin's office he motioned for me to sit on a chair in front of his desk, then told me, quite simply, to talk about myself, pressing the tips of his fingers together and watching me very closely. He was the leader of one of the foremost neuroscientific research groups in the world.

And what I saw there was yet another potential avenue for a young doctor with an enthusiasm for neuroscience; another way of using and exploring knowledge. I was introduced to an academic who had once been a physician, but left medicine for pure science because he found the former too boring. 'The good days were far outnumbered by the bad days', he told me of his clinical practice, and he hadn't worked as a doctor for twenty-five years. 'But to do science you have to have a kind of arrogance', he cautioned me, 'you have to believe that you can take on Nature and beat the truths out of her. You have to have a fire inside you that wouldn't give you peace until you have cracked a problem.'

I came away from that visit with the realization that I had no fire in my belly to 'defeat' nature in the way I'd been told was necessary for an elite scientific career. Science in that pure form was too focused; when the world around me seemed brimming with a diversity of experience I wanted instead to find a way to live with it, and try to understand that small part of it which related to me. From Maryland I returned to Scotland, and to the third part of my journeys.

Another friend, Donald Johnson, now an anaesthetist in Western Australia, was then working as a junior surgeon in a small hospital in the Scottish Highlands—one with just two wards, and a tiny emergency department. He thought I might learn as much about medicine there as I had on the other placements, but in addition would actually be of use: taking blood from patients, filing paperwork, holding retractors in the operating theatre. And so it proved—I discovered my love of medicine as a generalist.

Through giving up on the idea of mastery of one organ or disease, the horizons of possibility seemed to expand. East Africa and Bethesda had each taught something of the many ways of practising medicine, and primed me for an immersion in what would be the next step in my training: hospital medicine as a junior doctor in the UK's NHS.

I've made many journeys since those ones as an undergraduate, and seen medical schools and hospitals all over the world. To West Africa, India, Greenland, Antarctica. I studied for a Masters in Remote Health Care, exploring the many ways that twenty-first-century medicine could be adapted to being practised hundreds or thousands of miles from any hospital. I lectured on the strange synergies between medicine and literature in New York and in Moscow. But these excursions were always brief, and I always came back to my general medical practice in Scotland.

There's a line in Shakespeare's *As You Like It* that speaks to the weariness of experience, as opposed to the pleasures of it: 'but it is a melancholy of mine own, compounded of many simples, extracted from many objects, and indeed the sundry contemplation of my travels, which, by often rumination, wraps me in a most humorous sadness.' There are times when the brevity of my travels, and the paucity of what I have achieved with them, 'wraps me in a most humorous sadness', and I regret having passed so much of my medical career in a simple community clinic, near Edinburgh's city centre, rather than in further, deeper, more expansive journeys. And there are times when that very rootedness, and the personal and professional relationships that have flourished, and the books I've written because of it, convince me that choosing a small practice rooted in one place is the most worthwhile path I could have taken.

*

Browne wrote little of the journeys he undertook as part of his own medical training, but one of the most famous passages of his prose meditates on the fruits of doing what Pascal said we were unable to do: sit quietly in a room, alone:

> I could never content my contemplation with those general pieces of wonder, the flux and reflux of the sea, the increase of Nile, the conversion of the Needle to the North; and therefore have studied to match and parallel those in the more obvious and neglected pieces of Nature, which without further travel I can do in the cosmography of my self; we carry with us the wonders we seek without us: There is all Africa and her prodigies in us; we are that bold and adventurous piece of nature, which he that studies wisely learns in a compendium, what others labour at in a divided piece and endless volume.[10]

Coleridge marked up this passage in his copy of *Religio Medici*, with a scribbled: 'This is the true characteristic of Genius—our destiny & instinct is to unriddle the world.'[11] But it seems to me that Browne here is the riddle—it's the mystery of his own humanity that he approaches with awe. He was content to travel short distances around Norfolk, and though he encouraged all his children to travel, was happy to remain home, and hear about those travels by letter. He's said to have left no great estate because of the sums he gave to each of the four that survived to adulthood, and which all used, in part, to journey on the European Continent. He instructs them to journey with an open mind, to be 'courteous and civil to all' and to put on a 'commendable boldness'.

He was ambitious too for their social mobility—his daughters married well, and Edward reached far higher than he did in the hierarchies of nobility which then (and still) govern the social and intellectual life of England. His attitude on the importance of travel not just to broaden the mind, but as a means of personal advancement, reminds me of something Boswell said about Dr Johnson.

> He talked with an uncommon animation of traveling into distant countries; that the mind was enlarged by it, and that an acquisition of dignity of character was derived from it. He expressed a particular enthusiasm with respect to visiting the wall of China. I catched it for the moment, and said I really believed I should go and see the wall of China had I not children, of whom it was my duty to take care. 'Sir, (said he,) by doing so, you would do what would be of importance in raising your children to eminence. There would be a luster reflected upon them from your spirit and curiosity. They would be at all times regarded as the children of a man who had gone to view the wall of China. I am serious Sir.'[12]

*

There was throughout Thomas Browne's life a pervasive sense of motion, of change, from the journeys of his youth, to the social mobility of which he was so conscious, to the travels he must have made into the lives and stories of his patients to have become so trusted and respected as a physician. There's one final aspect of his mobility I'd like to examine: his flights of the imagination.

Browne's short work *Museum Clausum* is not so much read today, but offers insight into his rarely seen sense of humour, and a hint at the intellectual enthusiasms that governed him even into old age. It was published posthumously, and must have been written at some time in the last decade of his life. It proposes a hypothetical 'sealed museum' of 'remarkable books, antiquities, pictures and rarities of several kinds, scarce or never seen by any man now living'.[13]

Browne was fond of counterfactuals, imagining, for example, how the history of Europe might have been had Alexander gone west to destroy Rome, instead of east to destroy Persia, and in the *Museum Clausum* he suggests a series of books, letters, and images that might similarly have transformed our understanding of the past and changed the reality of the world we inhabit. Among twenty listed books, he imagines the book of poetry Ovid might have written in the local, barbarian dialect of the Black Sea while in exile. He conjures on the page the potential impact of finding authentic travel accounts of the Carthaginians Hannibal and Hanno—the former as he journeyed into Italy with his elephants, and the latter down the west coast of Africa and perhaps around the Cape of Good Hope almost two millennia before Vasca da Gama. Browne wonders whether lost members of Hanno's fleet 'fell into the Trade Winds, and were carried over into the coast of America'.[14] He yearns for the lost book of Pytheas of Massalia, *Concerning the Ocean*, quoted by Scipio and Strabo, and which described reaching Europe's farthest habitable north, *Ultima Thule*—the first written account of the Britons. Though known well in antiquity, the book is now lost to scholarship. Of thirty-four pictures: a map of the Mediterranean sea bed; a moonlit portrait of a Persian battle of Tamerlane; an image of the great fire of Constantinople; an elephant dancing on a tight-rope; a painting of Julia Gonzaga, the beauty of Italy, 'flying away with her ladies half naked on horseback'[15] from the sack of her city by Barbarossa. Finally, among twenty-five 'antiquities and rarities' that Browne imagines, a love of imaginative travel is similarly prominent: some medals of Justinian left in remote India by those

Friars, mentioned in Procopius, who first brought silkworms and knowledge of sericulture into Europe; vegetable horns that, set in the ground, 'grow up like Plants about Goa'; the ink of the type of cuttlefish that Hippocrates claimed would cure hysteria; salt from the Sargasso Sea; the ring with which the Doge of Venice wedded the sea, pulled from the stomach of a fish.

When he wrote these words, Browne had, for the best part of forty years, scarcely left Norwich and its immediate surroundings. Its contents confirm that, while preoccupied with his patients, his wife, his children, study, and books, a great part of him had never stopped travelling; he enjoyed a perpetual intellectual mobility that was no less agile for being rooted to home.

One of Browne's greatest modern admirers was the Canadian physician William Osler, one of the founders of Johns Hopkins Hospital in Baltimore, and, like Browne, a man of faith (Osler contemplated becoming a clergyman before he decided on a career in medicine). Osler travelled widely, was honoured as equally in Oxford as he was in Baltimore, and in later life was awarded a baronetcy, but it's less remarked upon in his many biographies that he was buried with a copy of Browne's *Religio Medici.* Osler seems to have considered Browne's works a kind of travel guide for life, and in particular, a life in medicine. One of his addresses to aspiring physicians counselled:

> Sealed early of this tribe of authors, a student takes with him, as compagnons de voyage, lifelong friends whose thoughts become his thoughts and whose ways become his ways. Mastery of self, conscientious devotion to duty, deep human interest in human beings—these best of all lessons you must learn now or never: and these are some of the lessons which may be gleaned from the life and from the writings of Sir Thomas Browne.[16]

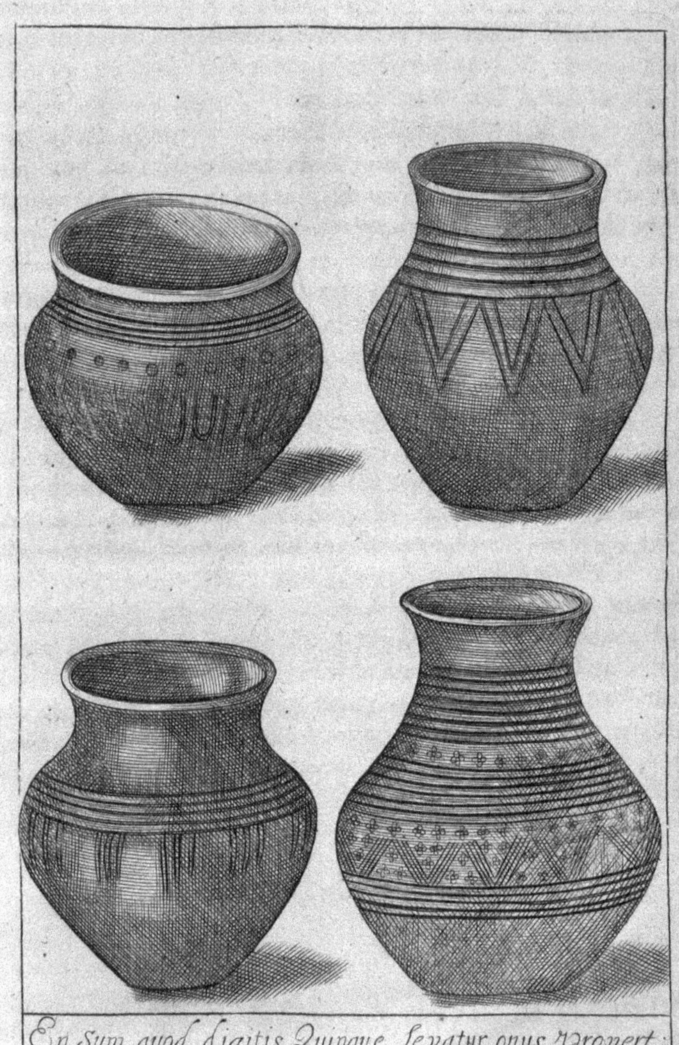

En Sum quod digitis Quinque Levatur onus Propert:

8

MORTALITY

Sir Thomas Browne is neither more nor less than the very prose-laureate of death ... And yet it may be said of [his works], that, like heaven itself, there is no death there.

Alexander Whyte
Sir Thomas Browne and his 'Religio Medici': An Appreciation (1898).

[Physicians] daily behold examples of mortality, and of all men least need artificial memento's, or coffins by our bed side, to mind us of our graves.
Urn Burial

Among the Stone Age collections of the National Museum of Scotland, you'd be forgiven for thinking we should name it instead the 'Bone Age'. Vitrine after vitrine of spears, arrowheads, scrapers, amulets, made not of stone, but of bone. From Shetland to Mull to the basin of the Tweed: beads, needles, and mattocks; arrowheads, spears, and cups; all carved from the bones of animals that were hunted, farmed, or found washed up on the beach. We know their age thanks to the carbon these animals breathed and ate.

In the museum, a ritual division between human and animal bones is maintained: the former, with their urns and accessories, are accorded deeper respect and displayed in an adjacent space. There are the remains of a dismembered boy from the Hebrides, inexplicably buried with the quartered carcasses of cattle and sheep. There is a series of children's skulls from a cave east of Inverness, found arranged on the cave floor in such a way that those heads seemed to have been suspended for a time from its ceiling as ghoulish stalactites. And from the Forth estuary, the urns and cists of long-dead folk buried four thousand years ago or more. In a series of pits along that coast were found decapitated heads from who knows what ritual of commemoration, propitiation, or retribution. Family groups interred in a huddle; a man under a coracle of leather; jars of cremated ashes.

Standing in contemplation of these exhibits, the first emotion that surfaced in me was one of recognition: of human lives, families, and livelihoods, with their accompanying necklaces, hammers, and axes. In the span of life on Earth, four thousand years figures as almost nothing at all—less than two hundred generations. But almost as soon as that sensation of fraternity appeared, it seemed to collapse under a weight of strangeness. These people knew the same hills and beaches that I walk on with my own children. But their world was a distant, preliterate one of bone and earthenware, forest and shellfish, of leather and, for the wealthiest, bronze. A world where you might lay a loved one to rest on a bed of quartzite and oxhide, where you might sever the head of a child, and lower it into a pit.

*

The ashes of an adult human weigh just two or three kilogrammes, the weight of a newborn baby. 'How the bulk of a man should sink into so few pounds of bones and ashes', wrote Browne, 'may seem strange unto any who considers not its constitution.'[1] The occasion for the essay in which he writes this, *Urn Burial*, was the unearthing of some Anglo-Saxon urns from a Norfolk field. For a sizeable proportion of Browne's admirers, it's his finest work—published in 1658, in his fifty-third year. He opens the essay considering how apposite the theme of mortality is to practitioners of medicine: '[T]o preserve the living, and make the dead to live, to keep men out of their urns, and discourse of humane fragments in them, is not impertinent unto our profession.' As a doctor, his many objects of study include life and death, and his profession offers him daily examples of the proximity of the latter. The very vicinity of death makes the physician the ideal commentator on what is an eternal theme of the human predicament. Medicine, too, is a profession that inures its practitioners, through habitual contact, to the more gruesome or melancholy aspects of death. Mortality is a theme never out of fashion, which may be another reason why this essay remains his most famous, more recognizable even than *Religio Medici*. Jorge Luis Borges loved it, quoting it with a frequency second only to *Vulgar Errors*.

It is customary to describe *Urn Burial* as one of the most glorious, ornate, and baroque essays of its period, indeed, of all English literature. That Browne thought the urns were Roman would perhaps be fatal to a lesser writer, but the error doesn't detract from the grandiloquence of the inspiration they offer him, or ultimately the merit of his reflections. Though the essay's ostensible purpose is a description of the urns, his prose and arguments range unrestrained over many other objects of his curiosity and learning. Its five parts mirror the five sections of its companion essay, *The Garden of Cyrus* (which concerns forms and symmetry in botany, and by extension, all nature), which themselves reflect the five states of being—matter, plants, animals, human, and spirit. It is almost as if Browne wished death and new life to sit adjacent on the page.

He seemed to want to demonstrate the fraternity of life and death, their interdependence.

The discovery of the urns prompts Browne at first to lead the reader through the funerary practices of biblical and Classical antiquity, and what he has heard of death traditions around the world. The specifics of those Norfolk urns are then described, with what he knows of funereal rituals in nearby Scandinavia during Roman times. The Egyptian pyramids are invoked both as magisterial monuments and as evidence of the vanity and futility of hoping for everlasting fame, then he comments on the conceit that nonsensically leads people to decorate mausoleums for the dead with greater care than they take over homes for the living. There are discussions of inscriptions and epitaphs, timing and positioning of interments, grave goods and yew trees. Browne considers, then discards, reincarnation ('A great part of antiquity contented their hopes of subsistency with a transmigration of their souls'[2]) then Buddhistic annihilation ('Others rather than be lost in the uncomfortable night of nothing were content to recede into the common being, and make one particle of the public soul of all things'[3]). The prose of his essay builds in complexity and majesty—the customary comparison is that of organ music—until at the end of Part V he reaches his climax, which is oddly brief and even anticlimactic: faith in bodily resurrection, and triumphal entry into a life eternal through Christ.

The brevity of his conclusion makes it clear that life everlasting doesn't interest Browne nearly as much as his foregoing contemplations of death on Earth. Eternal life, for him, is almost beyond conjecture, and so not worthy of substantial consideration; as he writes earlier in the same essay, 'a dialogue between two infants in the womb concerning the state of this world, might handsomely illustrate our ignorance of the next.'[4] With that, the matter appears to have been satisfactorily settled, and he goes back to what he knows, can read, and observe. He seems almost to tap us on the shoulder, to say 'stop, look at this wonder', only to rush us past, leading us on into ever-greater mysteries.

The following passage from the final section of *Urn Burial* may yet survive in quotation long after the rest of Browne's prose has been forgotten:

> But the iniquity of oblivion blindly scatters her poppy, and deals with the memory of men without distinction to merit of perpetuity. Who can but pity the founder of the Pyramids? Herostratus lives that burnt the Temple of Diana, he is almost lost that built it; Time has spared the Epitaph of Adrian's horse, confounded that of himself. In vain we compute our felicities by the advantage of our good names, since bad have equal durations; and Thersites is like to live as long as Agamemnon.* Who knows whether the best of men be known? or whether there be not more remarkable persons forgot, than any that stand remembered in the known account of time? Without the favour of the everlasting register, the first man had been as unknown as the last, and Methuselah's long life had been his only chronicle. Oblivion is not to be hired: The greater part must be content to be as though they had not been, to be found in the Register of God, not in the record of man.[5]

As a survey of burial practices as well as an exposition of the idiocy inherent in any expectation of enduring fame, *Urn Burial* points out that the ashes and urns of those buried anonymously in his Norfolk field have outlasted great monuments built above the Earth by more vainglorious men. 'Gravestones tell truth scarce

* Herostratus was the arsonist of the Temple of Artemis in Ephesus; the epitaph of Emperor Hadrian's horse Borysthenes survives; Thersites was a Greek at Troy, infamous for carping criticism of Agamemnon (and slain by Achilles). Browne is noting wryly that ignominy is as likely to offer immortality as nobility.

forty years. Generations pass while some trees stand, and old families last not three oaks.'[6] But there's another element of his essay on mortality that, though expounded less explicitly, seeps onto every page. Grief. By the time of *Urn Burial*'s publication, Browne's wife Dorothy had given birth to ten children, and the couple had suffered the deaths of five of them: Dorothy (1649–1652), Frances (1650–1651), Charles (1665–1672), and twins James and Richard (born August 1656 and lived for two months and fourteen months respectively).[7] Though his supposed subject is the burial urns, and by extension human frailty and mortality, I've always felt that the essay is, at its heart, about bereavement. Browne's principal theme is frail humanity's perpetual search for consolation, in the certain knowledge of oblivion.

*

To the right of the altar in an old church in Bologna stands a series of sculptures baked from clay. They are more than five hundred years old: six figures arrayed around a dead Christ, who lies supine on the floor, head on a tasselled cushion. Together they make up the *Compianto su Cristo morto* by Niccolò dell'Arca. A 'compianto' is a lamentation, and the fired earth of their terracotta—so much more vivid than marble or limestone—recalls the clays of Genesis from which human beings are moulded, and to which they must all return. The manifest devastation of anguish and woe have rarely been given such dramatic physical form. The figures are the Madonna, Mary Magdalene, Mary of Clopas, the apostle John, Joseph of Arimathea, and Mary mother of James—each expresses a moment of profound horror, frozen at the moment of realizing Jesus is dead.

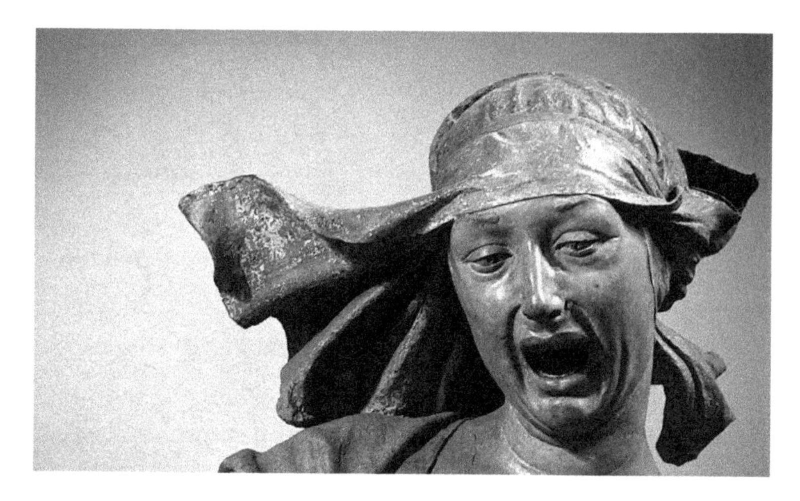

I mention them here because of Browne's connection with that part of Italy. The sculptures were already almost two centuries old when Browne studied in nearby Padua, and though we don't know for certain that he visited Bologna, it is likely that he did, and if so he may well have seen them. Bologna was under the Papal States at the time, while Padua was part of Venice; as a consequence the latter was a relative haven of intellectual freedom (to which Galileo notoriously fled). Yet there was relatively close intellectual traffic between the two university cities, and Browne, as a follower of Ulisse Aldrovandi (the naturalist who laid out the botanical gardens of Bologna), must have wanted to see the home city of his hero.[†] Browne was fascinated by gardens as emblematic of harmonies in nature—something he revisits repeatedly through his later book *Garden of Cyrus*.

[†] Aldrovandi died the year Browne was born. Aldrovandi's most famous work, the *Monstrorum Historia* or *History of Monsters*, would have resonated with Browne's fascination with generation and mutation, but the book wasn't published until 1642, long after Browne had left northern Italy and was established in Norwich.

The old church is *Santa Maria della Vita* (St Mary of Life). I went once to see Niccolò dell'Arca's sculptures with my children, when they were old enough that I thought they might begin to understand something of their power. There were beggars at the entranceway, a young woman in the front pew was weeping. Even approaching from the back of the church, the message of those sculpted faces was universal and unmistakable, eloquent across five centuries. Already hushed by the thick church silence, the children moved closer to me for comfort and, by the time I sat down, all three were scrambling for my lap. It seemed fitting that in a church dedicated to new life there should be such a devastating enactment of the perennial shock of death. My wife said later that she didn't feel the horror so acutely, perhaps because, with her Italian Catholic upbringing, she knew instinctively that the next chapter in Jesus's story, after the lamentation, is the resurrection. But though the resurrection must have been central to the sculptor's faith, I could think only of the authentic grief portrayed by his models, and how often he must have seen parents grieve children dead of fever, adult daughters dead of childbirth, adult sons dead of military conscription and injury. That period of European history knew death in a way Browne still knew it, but which has been vanquished in our own age not just by medicine and vaccination, but by the institutions of hospital and hospice.

The main church of Santa Maria della Vita was built in the later seventeenth century—only an extant side chapel stood at the time Browne visited this part of Italy. Nearby was its namesake hospital—*Ospedale della Vita,* the Hospital of Life—established in the 1200s for the care of pilgrims and the poor. Another local hospital was dedicated to the care of prisoners and those condemned to death: the *Ospedale della Morte*—the Hospital of Death.

For centuries, these two hospitals ran side by side, Life and Death, each a stone's throw from the city's university.

Browne arrived in Italy directly from Montpellier—a seat of medical education so ancient its curriculum was still largely inspired by Arab learning, and famous for the study of botany. Browne's tutor there, George Scharpe, was an itinerant Scotsman who later died in Bologna. But the fact that Browne decided to travel on into Italy from France, rather than go directly to Leiden or home to England, suggests that he sought deeper, newer understandings of healing than what was then considered old-fashioned Arab learning. It seems that his intention was to fuse the acquisition of knowledge of life as manifest in gardens, with a knowledge of death as it is displayed in the dissection room.

*

I had travelled down to Bologna from Padua, not principally for the terracotta sculptures, but to see Bologna's anatomy halls. The Edinburgh medical school I trained in owes a distant debt to both cities through what was, in the seventeenth century, their characteristic alloy of botany and anatomy.

A few years after Browne's Italian studies that amalgam was first carried to Scotland by Andrew Balfour, a young physician from Fife, born in 1630, who studied medicine first at St Andrews. But Balfour felt the need of further Continental education and journeyed, like Browne, to the north of Italy. It was thanks to Balfour that the practice of human dissection was taken back from the Po Valley to the Forth Valley, and that Edinburgh's first botanical gardens, for the education of physicians, apothecaries and surgeons, was laid out in the city. Balfour established the gardens on soil adjacent to a churchyard, with earth that had long been used for burial. He must have been conscious that in his choice of location he was choosing to pair death with vegetable and medicinal life; charnel house with glasshouse; grave with garden, just as Browne had with his *Urn Burial* and *Garden of Cyrus* just over a decade before (the garden was established in 1670).

Edinburgh's medicinal botanical gardens have moved twice since Balfour first paced them out in the later seventeenth century. The soil of his original garden is now compressed under the tonnes of brick that make up the southbound platforms of Edinburgh's principal railway station. Whenever I've taken the train from Edinburgh to London, or for that matter, Browne's home town of Norwich, I've passed a plaque that commemorates that hidden garden. To the sound of diesel engines, train-guard whistles, and tannoy announcements, I've hurried past, vaguely conscious of the almost-forgotten soil metres beneath my feet. Since the opening of the Channel Tunnel, the steel lines that overlay it now stretch all the way to France, and to Italy.

*

Though the principal aim of medicine must be the relief of human suffering, I wouldn't disagree with those who consider it the art of postponing death. Browne's introduction to *Urn Burial* again: 'to preserve the living, and make the dead to live, to keep men out of their urns, and discourse of humane fragments in them, is not impertinent unto our profession.' But 'make the dead to live'? The raising of Lazarus is one of Browne's recurring themes, but I don't think he meant this literally. He believed that there would be a bodily resurrection, but approached his theme also in the metaphorical sense that as an antiquarian he wished to bring vitality and deepened appreciation to his impressions of the past, to better inform his choices as to how to live. This can be done as well among the ancient bones of the basement of the National Museum of Scotland, as among recently unearthed urns in Norfolk. But beyond his discussion of antiquities, Browne must have been thinking of his work postponing death at the bedsides of the sick.

I was taught to diagnose death by shining a light into the glazed eyes of my patients before they'd even had a chance to get cold, in order to reassure myself there was no hint of pupillary contraction. I was then to lay a stethoscope on their chests until I was sure the heart and lungs were silent. I was to ask family members, or nursing staff, for an approximate time of death, but was never expected to associate it with the revolutions of celestial bodies as Browne did, nor ponder like him as to whether the intricate clockwork of human physiology runs down in sympathy with the moment it was wound up. Browne contemplated this phenomenon, of death on one's birthday, in his late work *Letter to a Friend*:

> in persons who outlive many years, and when there are no less than 365 days to determine their lives in every year, that the first day should mark the last, that the tail of the snake should return into its mouth precisely at that time, and that they should wind up upon the day of their nativity, is indeed a remarkable coincidence, which, though astrology has taken witty pains to solve, yet has it been very wary in making predictions of it.[8]

It's as if he had a sense that his own death would occur on his birthday.

It has always surprised me how little Browne wrote about his own life and health, barely mentioning his day-to-day medical practice. Perhaps his attention soars with his prose too loftily over the personal idiosyncrasies of medical case studies, slipping with ease away from the dirt and disease of the clinic, and up into universals. But there are moments in the historical record when his professional work shines through. A record of the Mayor's Court of Norwich dated from 1675 records the decision that two aldermen should approach Browne to discuss the eye condition suffered by one John Baliston, and ask Browne in particular about the prognosis.[9] There is a mid-seventeenth-century letter in the Norwich Records office, from Elizabeth Rous to her father Thomas Knyvett of Ashwellthorpe, in which Elizabeth encourages her father not give in to his ill health. Elizabeth adds, 'I hope docter browne will find both the cause and remedie.'[10]

When glimpses of medical encounters do appear in Browne's own hand, they're often among his correspondence. One of the most moving descriptions of a doctor–patient relationship occurs in *A Letter to a Friend*, when Browne describes the palliative care of a young man called Robert Loveday. It is crammed with Browne's characteristic wonderings: whether the waning moon or ebbing tide bring on men's deaths, whether hour of conception is related to time of death, how an 'old Italian' tutor told him death came more easily when the moon was falling from its meridian, whether ease of birth translates into difficulty dying. With regard to the latter, Loveday's death was so easy, Browne writes, 'that we might justly suspect his birth was of another nature, and that some *Juno* sat cross-legged at his Nativity', as she was said to have done at the birth of Hercules.

For Browne, life constituted a magnificent cathedral of mystery, shadowed and intricate, and the reader has the sense of him gladly setting out to explore it on our behalf. His writings offer no flood-light of illumination: in an age of such darkness, he seems content to leave much of it obscure. But using only the torch of his intellect, he beckons us to explore it with him little by little, as he was able.

*

As a general practitioner, one of my roles is to help those who wish to die at home achieve their ambition, and do whatever I can to keep them out of hospital. In a quarter century of practice I've sat with many for whom death is close, aiming not for Lazarus-like miracles, but for the relief of the suffering that is so often attendant on dying. In their final weeks, or days, or hours, some people become increasingly resolute, some become fearful, some become tranquil as if beatified, while yet others become irascible and cantankerous. In discussing death's approach, the *Letter* provides one of the most vivid examples of recognition across the centuries, when Browne discusses exactly those transformations in the personality of the dying that I've so often noticed myself.

> In this deliberate and creeping progress unto the grave, [Loveday] was somewhat too young, and of too noble a mind, to fall upon that stupid symptom observable in divers persons near their journeys end, and which may be reckoned among the mortal symptoms of their last disease; that is, to become more narrow minded, miserable and tenacious, unready to part with any thing when they are ready to part with all, and afraid to want when they have no time to spend.[11]

He reminds me of all those mild-mannered patients I've known whose tempers have grown shorter in proportion to the time they have left. 'The long habit of living makes mere men more hardly to part with life.'

So Loveday enjoyed a peaceful death. It struck Browne that one so young might be expected to inveigh against the illness that consumed him, even against his own mortality. But Browne's own experience (and perhaps the deaths of his children) had by then led him to believe otherwise—it is the young, who have least experience of life, who seem most ready to relinquish it. 'His willingness to leave this world about that age, when most men think they may best enjoy it, though paradoxical unto worldly ears, was not strange unto mine, who have so often observed, that many, though old, oft stick fast unto the world, and seem to be drawn like *Cacus's Oxen*, backward, with great struggling and reluctancy unto the grave.'[‡] This ability to illuminate paradox and demonstrate contrasting perspectives is characteristic of his thinking.

I am fortunate to live in a society where the deaths of children and young people are so unusual that a general practitioner working outside of paediatric hospital cannot comment with great experience on Browne's observation. But I observe that Loveday's reconciliation to death was to be admired not only for the way it acted to minimize his own suffering, and that of his family, but because it seemed to demonstrate a more virtuous mode of being. In his emphasis on the easy deaths of the young it's not difficult to see Browne reaching for consolation—so many of his own children died before reaching adulthood.

The path of virtue is difficult, he says: 'funambulous', in one of his more beautiful coinages (like an ant picking its way along a filament, or a tightrope walker). 'Tread softly and circumspectly in this funambulous track, and narrow path of goodness: pursue virtue virtuously', he writes. Ultimately the *Letter* is not so much a meditation on Loveday's death, as a guide book for life. We should aim to live so well as to have many wet eyes around our graves.

‡ *Cacus* was an ogre of classical mythology, who dragged oxen backwards in order to deceive Hercules as to their whereabouts.

For this we should avoid becoming too wealthy, because riches sweeten our deaths for those who might gather at our gravesides. His perspective is almost Buddhist in its acceptance; it is better to *content* oneself with death, than to actively yearn for it: 'Life may make us wish for death, but a virtuous one to rest in it.' Our mortality is not the end of us, but it is an end to the constant struggle to avoid sin. It is 'the horizon and isthmus between this life and a better, and the death of this world but as nativity of another'.

*

Towards the end of his life, Charles Darwin famously turned his thoughts towards the biology and habits of earthworms, as if conscious that the elements of which he was composed would shortly become food for them. Browne too wrote that he hoped to be as 'wholesome a morsel to the worms as any'.[12] His own death in 1682 was described by Thomas Townshend: 'Sir Thomas Browne is dead, and as he lived in an even temper without deep concern with how the world went, and was therein very happy so he died like a wise old philosopher.' As for his illness,

> He fell ill on Saturday, like a fever. All the physicians in town came to him, he understood the business himself and said he had a pain cross his stomach that nothing could remove, that he must die, and would take nothing neither physic nor cordial, but with all quietness and Christian meekness died yesterday, and is now pronounced a great and happy man in his life and death.[13]

And what of his children who, beyond his books, were his best hope of an enduring legacy? Of the five of his children that survived childhood, one was to die as a young man in battle: his favourite son Thomas, who had joined the navy. Many years before his death, Browne had written of his admiration for those who meet their ends with equanimity, and in particular those who die for a military cause: 'I honour any man that contemns it', he wrote of death,[§] 'nor can I highly love any that is afraid of it: this makes me naturally love a soldier, and honour those tattered and contemptible regiments that will die at the command of a sergeant.'[14] Thomas Browne the younger (born 1646) was killed in a sea battle against the Dutch (probably the Battle of Texel, August 1673), and his father's subsequent feelings about the waste of life perpetuated by war is one of the few occasions in which irritation appears amongst his writings.

Of the four children that survived him, his eldest son Edward (born in 1643) was the one that, as I've already described, reached greatest fame in London, as a physician traveller, and as courtier and Fellow of the Royal Society. Edward had one son, named Thomas, who died in 1711 just three years after Edward. The daughters that survived into adulthood were Anne (born 1647), Betty (born 1648), and Mary, the youngest (born in 1653).

By the 1720s, all of Browne's descendants were dead. Had he known how briefly his line would continue beyond his own death, I think he would have been sanguine. 'There is no antidote against the opium of time', he wrote, 'which temporally considers all things; our Fathers find their graves in our short memories, and sadly tell us how we may be buried in our survivors.'[15]

*

Of the nameless and numberless times that trace elements among human remains must have cycled through human, animal, and

§ Browne used 'contemn' rather as we might use 'contempt', but as a verb—a modern translation might be 'I honour any man that holds [death] in contempt.'

botanical re-embodiments, Browne had this to say, in his first published work *Religio Medici*:

> Now for the walls of flesh, wherein the soul does seem to be immured before the resurrection, it is nothing but an elemental composition, and a fabric that must fall to ashes. 'All flesh is grass' is not only metaphorically, but literally true, for all those creatures we behold are but the herbs of the field, digested into flesh in them, or more remotely carnified in ourselves. Nay, further, we are what we all abhor, anthropophagi and cannibals, devourers not only of men, but of ourselves; and that not in an allegory, but a positive truth; for all this mass of flesh which we behold came in at our mouths; this frame we look upon hath been upon our trenchers. In brief, we have devoured ourselves.[16]

This was written at just thirty years of age; Browne's imagination had already expanded into a realization that the ceaseless churn of elements essential to living bodies, through different 'carnifications' of life, had continued throughout the world's history. Earth's age, though, he pictured at just a few thousand years—about the age of those urns and skulls I've examined in the National Museum of Scotland.

He thought he was living near the end of days, but when he chose to summon an image of the changing face of the Earth and project it far into the future, he singled out our own age: 'And surely, he that has taken the true altitude of things, and rightly calculated the degenerate state of this age, is not like to envy those that shall live in the next, much less three or four hundred years hence, when no man can comfortably imagine what face this world will carry.'[17] To read Browne is to be reminded of impermanence and the implacability of time, and to have our gaze redirected to the revelation that each of us, no matter our longevity, is permitted only a glimpse of life. Like sparks from a perpetual fire that are extinguished within moments of ignition we flash into being, between irrecoverable depths of time past and eternities of what is to come. I too cannot 'comfortably imagine' what the world will be like four centuries from my own time, but Browne reassures me that I should busy myself with what I *can* begin to understand, and what I can *do*.

*

The saddest graveyards I ever saw were in India's Himachal Pradesh, in the hill stations built by the ruling class of the British Raj. Women and men who'd died of injuries, of fever, of the complications of childbirth, all buried in earth they believed (however erroneously) was theirs to rule, and who might have been expected to be better remembered. Many graves less than a century old were cracked and broken, trash had been tipped into their sanctuaries, some of the most substantial monuments had been used as toilets. They reminded me of something Browne's biographer, Samuel Johnson, said of the graves of Scottish kings in Iona: 'The graves are very numerous, and some of them undoubtedly contain the remains of men who did not expect to be so soon forgotten.'[18] But for Browne, all any of us can ever expect is to be forgotten; we must seek the worth of our work in life, not in memorials after death. 'In vain we hope to be known by open and visible conservatories', he wrote of the Norfolk urns, 'the man of God lives longer without a tomb than any by one, invisibly interred by angels.'[19]

Browne's point is that all graveyards are in their way sad, and beyond the succour they might offer the living, faintly ridiculous. From his perspective, we're here for what we can offer others (and

God). When we die, we might as well be buried in a mass grave as be the dedicatee of a Pyramid. ''Tis all one to lie in St *Innocents* Church-yard, as in the sands of Egypt: Ready to be any thing, in the ecstasy of being ever, and as content with six foot as the Moles of *Adrianus*.'[**,20]

Elsewhere Browne contemplated the 'error' of Adam and Eve by introducing sin, corruption, and death into humanity. 'Our ends are as obscure as our beginnings',[21] he wrote, and each of us are obliged to take our minuscule part in the cycles of life and death. Because of that error in the Garden of Eden, our lives are briefer, but for Browne they must also be richer.

*

It's traditional in any discussion of Browne's death to conclude with a story of his own grave and its disturbances. The man who wrote, 'But who knows the fate of his bones, or how often he is to be buried?', was first interred in his local church, but, just over a century later, his grave was opened and his skull stolen. It was then sold by the church sexton and ended up in a private collection of oddities, then on the shelves of the local hospital museum. It wasn't until the 1920s that the skull was reunited with his bones, and reburied.

The grave plate on Browne's coffin was found to have a Latin inscription:

> *Amplissimus Vir Thomas Browne Miles Medicinæ D. Annis Natus 77 Denatus 19 Die Mensis Octobris Anno D. 1682 hoc. Loculo indormiens Corporis Spagyrici pulvere plumbum in aurum convertit.'*

** 'the moles of Adrianus' is the elaborate mausoleum of the emperor Hadrian, now underneath the castle Sant'Angelo in Rome.

Which, according to an 1869 edition of Religio Medici, is best translated as:

> The very distinguished man, Sir Thomas Browne, Knight, Doctor of Medicine, aged 77 years, who died on the 19th of October, in the year of our Lord 1682, sleeping in this coffin of lead, by the dust of his alchemic body, transmutes it into a coffer of gold.[22]

Browne, then, was seen by those who buried him as a kind of alchemist, and just as he turned everyday observations into glittering insights when alive, so his 'alchemic' body had become transformed, from the lead of earthly life, into the gold of eternity.

Decemb 2 1679

In the name of God Amen. I Thomas Browne Knight and Dr of Physick of the citty of Norwich do make this my last will and testament. Inprimis I give and bequeath unto my dear wife Dame Dorothie Browne all my Lands houses and tenements all my bonds bills mouvables, money plate Jewells and all my goods whatsoever thereby to have a provision for her self and make a decent maintenance and portions for my deare daughters Elizabeth Browne and Frances Browne Excepting such Lands and tenements as were assigned and made over unto my sonne Edward Browne upon marriage and to bee entred upon by one after my decease. Of this I appoynt and make my wife Dame Dorothie Browne my sole Executrix and give her power to sell all houses all lands my goods mouvables mony plate Jewells and all goods valuable whatsoever for the provision of her self and of my daughters Elizabeth and Frances Browne and for the payment of my debts Legacies and charitable gifts [illegible] with she is fully acquainted and trust I doubt not performe my will therein. And if it shall please god that my wife Dame Dorothie should dye before mee then I make my daughters Elizabeth and Frances Browne my Executrices and give them the same power in my estate as I have before given unto my wife Dame Dorothie. This is my last will and testament which I have writt with my owne hand and confirmed it with my hand and seale.

witnesses

George [illegible]

Anthony Mingay

Aug: Briggs Junr

Thomas Browne

A CONCLUDING LETTER TO DR BROWNE

Dear Dr Browne,

I set out in this book with an image in mind of an alchemist's laboratory, and the intention to create a kind of distillation of your life and works rather than an orthodox biography. Just as the author of your grave plate wondered if your dust might transform the lead of your coffin into gold, I wondered if it might be possible to render something of the value of your legacy through a kind of alchemical process. Into a flask or crucible I intended to throw some reflections on the great themes of your life as I saw them with some of my favourite passages from your books then, with a sprinkling of others' words—Johnson to Coleridge, Thoreau to Woolf, Preston to Barbour—bubble the mixture together, to see what vapours might arise. But I'm not sure if that's entirely the best description of what I've achieved. Instead it feels more as if I've spent my time striking the dull grey iron of my own brain against the glinting flint of your prose to see what scattered sparks might emerge. At a distance of three and a half centuries that flint seems old now, but it's still sharp, and for me at least has yielded many glimmers of insight.

One of those insights is that to approach this book through a prism of your qualities, through your ambiguity, humility, or piety, didn't fully convey the richness and strangeness of much of your work. And approaching it through what are your greatest and most resonant themes: vitality and mortality, generation and senescence, didn't offer a broad enough sense of your life as a man of your age. Though it conveyed the magnificence of some of your literary achievements, it spoke less to your personal biography and characteristic genius. To better elucidate those elements of your work, I had to explore your sense of rootedness in a place and time, the seventeenth century, and your mobility both socially and across the intellectual and geographical landscapes of your Europe, and your England. I sought to put on display the depth of your restless and pervasive curiosity, show how it animated your reading, your practice of medicine, your understanding of the world of nature—a world that absorbed and enthralled you. Your century was one of war both at home and abroad; wars that killed your son and soured relationships between neighbours and between rulers and ruled. That you wrote nothing of those conflicts but consistently pursued an even-handed, fair-minded attitude in your correspondence, your books, and your relationships with your patients, is something I find immensely admirable, and is a large part of why reading you remains such a pleasure today.

In looking at the misogyny evident in your own work, I've tried to bring out some of the assumptions that I see woven into the fabric of your society, and that unavoidably filtered everything that you read and wrote. In my own country, women now make up around 60 per cent of medical students, and two-thirds of general practitioners, but still less than 30 per cent of surgeons. Medicine, as in the rest of society, has made some progress in terms of discrimination on the basis of sex, but remarkably little progress in terms of ethnicity and social class.

It's clear that these distinctive prisms through which I've peered at your work have been to a certain extent artificial. Your perspective on death is inseparable from your reflections on generation and new life; that fierce awareness of mortality so on display in *Urn Burial* is intermingled with your piety; the ambiguity of your prose is a reflection of the humility of your attitude; your prejudices are inextricable from your age, context, and travels; your curiosity about the world and about humanity is interwoven with all of these themes, and more. I'm glad to have spent these months in your company, rereading your books and discovering new commentaries and new perspectives on your life and work.

'Bless me in this life with but peace of my conscience, command of my affections, the love of thy self and my dearest friends, and I shall be happy enough to pity Cæsar',[1] you wrote. A life well lived has rarely been drawn so succinctly. You offered the consolation of eternal return when you wrote 'All things began in order, so shall they end, and so shall they begin again',[2] implying that in the greatest, truest sense, there is really no death. We are all of us granted a berth on what you called the 'virtuous voyage'; 'let not disappointment cause despondency, nor difficulty despair ... expect rough seas, flaws, and contrary blasts.'[3] You asked us to judge one another by our generosity, not our riches, and to cherish wonder. 'Live like a neighbour unto death', you wrote, 'and think there is but little to come.'[4] There is no antidote against the opium of time.

Yours,

Dr Gavin Francis MBChB (Hons) FRCGP FRCPEd
Edinburgh, 2022

ENDNOTES

Sources unless otherwise specified are from Charles Sayle's 1904 edition of the complete works of Browne.

RM—Religio Medici
VE—Vulgar Errors/Pseudodoxia Epidemica
UB—Urn Burial/Hydriotaphia
GC—The Garden of Cyrus
LF—Letter to a Friend
MC—Museum Clausum

Chapter 1: Ambiguity

1. 'it preserves its…' UNESCO World Heritage https://whc.unesco.org/en/list/824/ accessed October 2021.
2. 'Generations pass…' UB ch. 5.
3. Johnson, Samuel. *The Life of Sir Thomas Browne* in 2nd edition of *Christian Morals*. London, 1756.
4. Bacon, Francis. *The Great Instauration* (Preface). London, 1620.
5. Woolf, Virginia. *The Elizabethan Lumber Room* in *The Common Reader*, pp. 61–73, New York, 1925 (Harcourt, Brace & Company).
6. 'You might read…' Whyte, Alexander. *Sir Thomas Browne and the Religio Medici: An Appreciation*. Edinburgh, 1898 (Oliphant Anderson & Ferrier).
7. 'I have no…' RM Bk 1 section 6.
8. 'We have reformed…' RM Bk 1 section 3.
9. 'He does not…' Whyte, Alexander. *Sir Thomas Browne and the Religio Medici: An Appreciation*. Edinburgh, 1898 (Oliphant Anderson & Ferrier).
10. 'But the mortalest…' VE Bk 1 ch. 6.
11. 'nor have we…' VE introduction.

12. 'but my humours...' Montaigne. *Essays* in *On the Education of Children* in *The Essays of Michel de Montaigne*, trans. Charles Cotton, ed. William Carew Hazlitt. London, 1877.
13. 'A trust - ...' Biss, Eula. *On Immunity*. London, 2016 (Fitzcarraldo).
14. 'Upon my first...' LF
15. 'He was at ease...' Jamieson, Kay Redfield. *An Unquiet Mind*. London, 1997 (Vintage).
16. 'For a laugh...' VE Bk 7 ch. 16.
17. Szirtes, George. *Sir Thomas Browne as Melville's Crack'd Angel*. Lecture delivered to the Thomas Browne Society at Dragon Hall, Norwich, Friday 19 October 2018.

Chapter 2: Curiosity

1. 'there was a real...' White, T.H. *The Sword in the Stone*. London, 1982 (Fontana).
2. 'there were galls...' Macdonald, Helen. 'The forbidden wonder of birds' nests and eggs'. *The Guardian*, 9 September 2017.
3. *The Diary of John Evelyn*, ed. William Bray. London, 1901 (M. Walter Dunne).
4. 'kept them in...' VE Bk 2 ch. 7.
5. 'Out of the...' VE Bk 3 ch. 26.
6. 'The world was...' RM Bk 1 section 13.
7. 'The world that I...' RM Bk 2 section 11.
8. 'Thus we are men...' RM Bk 1 section 36.
9. 'Thou hast curiously...' GC ch. 3.
10. 'the same attention...' see Coleridge, Samuel Taylor, quoted in Brinkley, Roberta (ed.). *Coleridge on the Seventeenth Century*. Durham, 1955 (North Carolina), p. 448.
11. 'it is of small...' Johnson, Samuel. *The Life of Sir Thomas Browne* in 2nd edition of *Christian Morals*. London, 1756.
12. 'from heaven...' RM Bk 1 section 19.
13. 'Thus the Devil...' RM Bk 1 section 19.

Chapter 3: Vitality

1. 'I think I have...' RM Bk 2 section 11.
2. 'As a doctor who...' Sebald, W.G. *The Rings of Saturn*. London, 2002 (Vintage).

3. 'half-sweet, half-painful...' Mann, Thomas. *The Magic Mountain*, trans. H.T. Lowe-Porter. London, 1927.
4. 'Such a vast...' from Browne's correspondence with his son.
5. Preston, Claire. *Thomas Browne and the Writing of Early Modern Science* Cambridge, 2005, p. 194.
6. 'wherein the leaves...' Letter to Henry Power, 1659 quoted in Killeen, Kevin. *Biblical Scholarship, Science and Politics in Early Modern England; Thomas Browne and the Thorny Place of Knowledge*. Farnham, 2009 (Ashgate).
7. '[T]here may be...' RM Bk 1 section 32.
8. 'this is that...' RM Bk 1 section 32.
9. 'eighth or tenth...' VE Bk 4 ch. 7 *Concerning Weight*.
10. Confer no relief...' VE Bk 4 ch. 7 *Concerning Weight*.
11. 'The great variety...' GC ch. 3.
12. 'Seeds found in...' GC ch. 3.
13. 'The relation of...' VE Bk 7 ch 16 *Of divers Other Relations*.
14. 'no material part' Aristotle *The Generation of Animals*.
15. 'In Nature there is...' Swammerdam, Jan, quoted in Carlson, E.A. *Mendel's Legacy—The Origin of Classical Genetics*. 2004 (Cold Spring Harbor, Cold Spring Harbor Laboratory Press).
16. 'although her production...' VE Bk 6 ch. 1.
17. 'The forms of things...' VE Bk 3 ch. 27 *Compendiously of sundry Tenents concerning other Animals, which examined, prove either false or dubious*.
18. 'water in the flask...' Miller, S. L., and Urey, H. C. (1959). Organic Compound Synthesis on the Primitive Earth. *Science*, 130(3370), 245–251.
19. 'and the moon gazed...' Shelley, Mary. *Frankenstein; Or, the Modern Prometheus*. London, 1818, ch. 4.
20. 'desired to learn...' Shelley, Mary. ch. 2.
21. 'I am a blasted...' Shelley, Mary. ch. 19.
22. 'A hundred million...' de Bergerac, Cyrano. *A voyage to the moon: with some account of the solar world. A comical romance*, trans. Samuel Derrick. London, 1753.
23. 'Love everything into...' Wilson, Edward, quoted in Seaver, George. *The Faith of Edward Wilson*. London, 1948.
24. 'Life is a pure...' UB ch. 5.
25. 'we are only...' RM Bk 1 section 34.
26. 'first we are...' RM Bk 1 section 34.

27. From Calvino, Italo. *Six Memos for the Next Millennium*. London, 2009 (Penguin), p. 52.

Chapter 4: Piety

1. Whitefoot, Rev John. *Minutes for the Life of Sir Thomas Browne* published as a preface to the *Posthumous Works*. London, 1722.
2. 'though in point of…' Among Browne's Commonplace Books, quoted in *Religio Medici, A Letter to a Friend, Christian Morals, Urn Burial, & Other Papers*. Boston, 1862 (Ticknor & Fields).
3. 'pray daily…' Among Browne's Commonplace Books, quoted in *Religio Medici, A Letter to a Friend, Christian Morals, Urn Burial, & Other Papers*. Boston, 1862 (Ticknor & Fields).
4. 'There is, as in…' RM Bk 1 section 18.
5. 'This is exceedingly…' see Coleridge, Samuel Taylor, quoted in Brinkley, Roberta (ed.). *Coleridge on the Seventeenth Century*. Durham, 1955 (North Carolina), p. 441.
6. 'As for those…' RM Bk 1 section 9.
7. 'one day lived…' LF.
8. see Thaler Alwin. 'Sir Thomas Browne and the Elizabethans'. *Studies in Philology* Vol. 28, No. 1 (Jan., 1931), 87–117 (31 pages).

Chapter 5: Humility

1. 'his modesty was…' Whitefoot, John. *Minutes for the Life of Sir Thomas Browne* published as a preface to the *Posthumous Works*. London, 1722.
2. ed. Charles Sayle, published 1904.
3. 'a library was…' see Coleridge, Samuel Taylor, quoted in Brinkley, Roberta (ed.). *Coleridge on the Seventeenth Century*. Durham, 1955 (North Carolina), p. 447.
4. 'I'm telling you…' Carlos Williams, William. *Old Doc Rivers* in *The Doctor Stories*. New York, 1984 (New Directions).
5. [The specialists] wear dark…' Helman, Cecil. *Suburban Shaman*, London, 2006 (Hammersmith Press).
6. 'Therefore, if we have…' Bacon, Francis. *Historia Ventorum*, London, 1622 (John Haviland).
7. 'They that are…' UB ch. 1.

8. 'Indeed what reason...' RM Bk 1 section 15.
9. 'The choice of the vernacular' Preston, Claire. *Thomas Browne and the Writing of Early Modern Science*. Cambridge, 2005.
10. 'Be substantially great...' LF.
11. 'Bless me in this...' RM Bk 2 section 15.
12. Letter from Browne to Edward.
13. Johnson, Samuel. *The Life of Sir Thomas Browne* in 2nd edition of *Christian Morals*. London, 1756.

Chapter 6: Misogyny

1. Zayas y Sotomayor, María de. *The Enchantments of Love: Amorous and Exemplary Novels*, trans. Patsy Boyer. University of California Press, 1990.
2. Barbour, Reid. *Sir Thomas Browne: A Life*. Oxford, 2013 (OUP), letter quoted from 1669, p. 386.
3. 'Hermaphrodites...' VE Bk 3 ch. 12 *Of the Phoenix*
4. 'The whole world...' RM Bk 2 section 9
5. 'As for the...' VE Bk 3 ch. 17 *Of hares*
6. 'very strange and...' VE Bk 1 ch. 1 *Of the causes of Common Errors*
7. Zevit, Z. 1. (2015). Was Eve made from Adam's rib—or his baculum? *Biblical archaeology review*, 41(5), 32–35.
8. 'That a man...' VE Bk 7 ch. 2 *That a man hath one rib less than a woman*
9. 'we might procreate...' RM Bk 2 section 9
10. 'raillery of contemporary...' Johnson, Samuel *The Life of Sir Thomas Browne* in 2nd edition of *Christian Morals* London, 1756.
11. 'He says he is...' Coleridge, Samuel Taylor quoted in Brinkley Roberta (ed.) *Coleridge on the Seventeenth Century*, Durham,1955 (North Carolina)
12. Sebald, WG *The Rings of Saturn* London 2002 (Vintage) P68-69
13. 'I am, I confess...' RM Bk 1 section 3
14. 1 Samuel 28:3.
15. 'I have ever believed...' RM Bk 1 section 30
16. 'Of all the delusions...' RM Bk 1 section 30
17. Kaveney, Roz. Thomas Browne: religion as passion and pastime, part 1. *Guardian* May 20, 2013
18. A Tryal of Witches at the Assizes Held at Bury St. Edmonds 1682, quoted in Barbour, Reid. *Sir Thomas Browne: A Life*. Oxford, 2013 (OUP).
19. Barbour, Reid. *Sir Thomas Browne: A Life*. Oxford, 2013 (OUP), p. 368.

20. VE Bk 4 ch. 6 *Of Swimming & Floating*
21. British Library Additional MS 36,988, 195v.

Chapter 7: Mobility

1. 'I have been...' RM Bk 2 section 1.
2. 'Ireland had...' Johnson, Samuel. *The Life of Sir Thomas Browne* in 2nd edition of *Christian Morals*. London, 1756.
3. 'melancholy accounts...' Boyle, Robert. *New experiments and observations touching cold, or, An experimental history of cold begun to which are added an examen of antiperistasis and an examen of Mr. Hobs's doctrine about cold.* London, 1665 (John Crook).
4. 'I, on my...' Thoreau, Henry David. *Walden*. Boston, 1854 (Ticknor & Fields).
5. 'it is interesting...' Strachey, L. *Literary Essays: Books and Persons*. London, 1922 (Chatto).
6. 'Tickets on this line...' Forster, E.M. *The Celestial Omnibus and other stories*. London, 1912 (Sidgwick & Jackson).
7. 'Those national repugnances...' RM Bk 2 section 1.
8. 'I wonder not...' RM Bk 2 section 1.
9. 'In our age...' Bartholin, Thomas. *On Medical Travel*. Copenhagen, 1674.
10. 'I could never...' RM Bk 1 section 15.
11. 'This is the true...' see Coleridge, Samuel Taylor, quoted in Brinkley, Roberta (ed.). *Coleridge on the Seventeenth Century*. Durham, 1955 (North Carolina).
12. 'He talked with...' Boswell, James. *Life of Johnson*. London, 1791.
13. 'remarkable books' MC—subtitle.
14. 'fell into the...' MC part 1 section 6.
15. 'flying away with...' MC part 2 section 20.
16. 'Sealed early...' Osler, W. 'Sir Thomas Browne' in *An Alabama Student and Other Biographical Essays*. London, 1929 (OUP).

Chapter 8: Mortality

1. 'How the bulk...' UB ch. 3.
2. 'A great part of...' UB ch. 4.
3. 'Others rather than...' UB ch. 4.
4. 'A dialogue between...' UB ch. 4.

5. 'But the iniquity...' UB ch. 5.
6. 'Gravestones tell truth...' UB ch. 5.
7. The details of these births and deaths are taken from Reid Barbour's biography of Browne.
8. 'in persons who outlive...' LF.
9. *Norfolk Record Office: NCR 16a/25.*
10. *Norfolk Record Office: KNY 775, 372×5.*
11. 'In this deliberate...' LF.
12. 'wholesome a morsel...' RM Bk 1 section 40.
13. Thomas Townshend quotation on the death of Browne—quoted in Barbour, Reid. *Sir Thomas Browne: A Life*. Oxford, 2013 (OUP), p. 466.
14. 'I honour any...' RM Bk 1 section 38.
15. 'There is no...' UB ch. 5.
16. 'Now for the walls...' RM Bk 1 section 37.
17. 'and surely, he...' LF.
18. 'The graves are...' Boswell, James. *The Journal of a Tour to the Hebrides with Samuel Johnson, LL.D.* London, 1785.
19. 'In vain we hope...' UB ch. 5.
20. 'tis all one...' UB ch. 5.
21. 'our ends are...' RM Bk 1 section 43.
22. 'The very distinguished...' see *RELIGIO MEDICI etc*, with Introduction & Notes by J. W. Willis Bund. London, 1869 (Sampson Low, Son, & Marston).

A Concluding Letter to Dr Browne

1. 'Bless me...' RM Bk 2 section 15.
2. 'All things began...' GC ch. 5.
3. 'let not disappointment...' LF.
4. 'live like a neighbour...' LF.

POSTHUMOUS

WORKS

Of the Learned

Sir *Thomas Browne*, Kt. M. D.

Late of NORWICH.

Printed from his Original *Manuſcripts*,

VIZ.

I. REPERTORIUM: Or, The Antiquities of the Cathedral Church of *NORWICH*.
II. An Account of ſome URNS, *&c.* found at *Brampton* in *Norfolk*, *Anno* 1667.
III. LETTERS between Sir *William Dugdale* and Sir *Thomas Browne*.
IV. MISCELLANIES.

To which is prefix'd his LIFE.

There is alſo added,
Antiquitates Capellæ D. Johannis Evangeliſtæ; *hodie Scholæ Regiæ* Norwicenſis. *Authore* Johanne Burton, A. M. *ejuſdem Ludimagiſtro.*

Illuſtrated with *Proſpects*, *Portraitures*, *Draughts* of *Tombs*, *Monuments*, &c.

LONDON:
Printed for W. MEARS, at the *Lamb* without *Temple Bar*, and J. HOOKE, at the *Flower-de-Luce* againſt *St. Dunſtan's* Church in *Fleetſtreet*.
MDCCXXIII. (*Price Six Shillings.*)

FURTHER READING

Charles Sayle's 1904 edition of Browne's complete works is available for free online, at www.gutenberg.org, and is the edition I own and used in the research for this book. Below are listed some other books that I've drawn on, been inspired by, or refer to.

Aldersey-Williams, Hugh. *The Adventures of Sir Thomas Browne in the 21st Century*. London, 2015 (Granta)

Barbour, Reid. *Sir Thomas Browne: A Life*. Oxford, 2013 (OUP)

Bartholin, Thomas. *On Medical Travel* Copenhagen, 1674

Brinkley, Roberta (ed.). *Coleridge on the Seventeenth Century*. Durham, 1955

Browne, Sir Thomas. *Religio Medici & Urne-Buriall*, eds. Greenblatt, Stephen, & Targoff, Ramie. New York, 2012 (NYRB)

Forster, E.M. *The Celestial Omnibus and Other Stories*. London, 1912 (Sidgwick & Jackson)

Hitchings, Christopher. *Samuel Johnson and Sir Thomas Browne*. PhD thesis submitted to UCL (2002)

Johnson, Samuel. *The Life of Sir Thomas Browne* from the 2nd edition of *Christian Morals*. London, 1756

Killeen, Kevin. *Biblical Scholarship, Science and Politics in Early Modern England; Thomas Browne and the Thorny Place of Knowledge*. Farnham, 2009 (Ashgate)

Killeen, Kevin. *Thomas Browne: Selected Writings*. Oxford, 2018 (OUP)

Peter, Martens. The Faiths of Two Doctors: Thomas Browne and William Osler. *Perspectives in Biology and Medicine*, Johns Hopkins University Press, Volume 36, Number 1, Autumn 1992, pp. 120–128, 10.1353/pbm.1993.0048

Preston, Claire. *Sir Thomas Browne: Selected Writings*. New York, 2003 (Routledge)

Preston, Claire. *Thomas Browne and the Writing of Early Modern Science* Cambridge, 2005 (Cambridge)

Sebald, W.G. *The Rings of Saturn*. London, 2002 (Vintage)

Szirtes, George. *Sir Thomas Browne as Melville's Crack'd Angel.* Lecture delivered to the Thomas Browne Society at Dragon Hall, Norwich, Friday 19 October 2018. Available through www.sirthomasbrowne.org.uk

Whitefoot, Rev. John. *Minutes for the Life of Sir Thomas Browne* published as a preface to the *Posthumous Works* London, 1722

Whyte, Alexander. *Sir Thomas Browne and the Religio Medici: An Appreciation.* Edinburgh, 1898 (Oliphant Anderson & Ferrier)

Woolf, Virginia. *The Elizabethan Lumber Room* in *The Common Reader,* pp. 61–73 New York, 1925 (Harcourt, Brace & Company)

ACKNOWLEDGEMENTS

With abundant gratitude to the many scholars without whose transporting works I would have been shipwrecked on the rocky outskirts of Browne's world, unable to visit its transformative heartlands and uplands.

> *Scholars are men of peace, they bear no arms, but their tongues are sharper than Actius's razor; their pens carry farther, and give a louder report than thunder.*

To Claire Preston, who noticed in my own book *Adventures in Human Being* an affection for Browne, and who as a consequence invited me to speak with her at the opening of an exhibition in celebration of Browne at London's Royal College of Physicians in January 2017. Her two books acknowledged here have in particular had a profound influence on the way I read and think about Browne.

To Kevin Killeen, whose scholarship and enthusiasm have been a boon. I'm grateful for the exchanges in which he has offered me advice, guidance, and references—in particular sharing with me more about the connections between William Osler and Browne, and more about Browne's quotidian medical practice. He has been unfailingly generous both about my approach to writing on Browne, and in suggestions to improve the text.

To Hugh Aldersey-Williams, whose *The Adventures of Sir Thomas Browne in the 21st Century* (2015) was a welcome introduction to Browne's relevance today, and whose enthusiasm and Brownean curiosity are an inspiration.

To Reid Barbour, whose *Sir Thomas Browne: A Life* (2013) allowed me to trace the contours of Browne's life with far more reliable texture than would otherwise have been possible. At first I felt awash in stories about Browne; by bringing together so many sources Barbour threw me a lifeline.

To Marion Catlin, an enthusiast of Browne who has done so much to promote Browne's memory not just in Norwich, but nationally and internationally, through her work to celebrate Browne Day on October 19, and through establishing and maintaining the site https://www.sirthomasbrowne.org.uk

To Kevin Faulkner of Norwich who spoke with me about the *spagyrical* and alchemical coffin-plate found in Browne's grave, about Paracelsus and Browne, and for his tireless efforts to celebrate and commemorate Browne's life.

To Charlotte Higgins for helping me to explore the many meanings of piety, *regere*, and εὐσεβεῖν.

To Marina Warner, for first asking if I'd consider writing a book about Browne, and for being such an enthusiastic supporter of the book as it evolved, as well as one of its first readers.

To Philip Davis and Jacqueline Norton, who have been generous and visionary editors of this OUP series. Their openness to my own idiosyncratic approaches to Browne's life and work have been most welcome.

Last of all I'd like to thank Dr Thomas Browne, for leaving at his death such a legacy of literary, medical, and intellectual riches. 'I instruct no man as an exercise of my knowledge, or with an intent rather to nourish and keep it alive in mine own head than beget and propagate it in his', he wrote. 'And, in the midst of all my endeavours, there is but one thought that dejects me, that my acquired parts must perish with myself, nor can be legacied among my honoured friends.'

This is one of the (few) cases in which Browne was in error. In opening one of his books, each of us becomes an 'honoured friend', and can benefit from the humanity and generosity, the vitality and curiosity, the humility and ease with ambiguity, so evident in this extraordinary man's life and in his work.

INDEX

Note: The index covers the main text but the endnotes only very selectively. An italic '*f*' following a page number denotes an illustration, 'n' alone indicates a footnote and n followed by a number, an endnote.